[ ~~~~~~~~~~~~~~~~ ce 1977, after spending six years in ge   .l practice and seven years in medical research. He writes the 'Doctor, Doctor' column in the *Guardian* on Saturdays, and has written three humorous books, *Doctor, Have You Got a Minute?*, *A Seaside Practice* and *Going Loco*, all published by Short Books. His other books for Sheldon Press include *Heart Attacks: Prevent and Survive*, *Living with Alzheimer's Disease*, *Overcoming Back Pain*, *Coping with Bowel Cancer*, *Coping with Heartburn and Reflux*, *Coping with Age-related Memory Loss*, *Skin Cancer: Prevent and Survive*, *How to Get the Best from Your Doctor*, *Coping with Kidney Disease* and *Osteoporosis: Prevent and Treat*.

# Overcoming Common Problems Series

*Selected titles*

A full list of titles is available from Sheldon Press,
36 Causton Street, London SW1P 4ST and on our website at
www.sheldonpress.co.uk

Overcoming Common Problems

# Coping Successfully with Prostate Cancer

## Second Edition

DR TOM SMITH

*For Joanna Moriarty and Fiona Marshall, of Sheldon Press, who have given me such great support and encouragement over more years than any of the three of us would like to disclose*

First published in Great Britain in 2002
Second edition 2010

Sheldon Press
36 Causton Street
London SW1P 4ST

British Library Cataloguing-in-Publication Data
A catalogue record for this book is available from the British Library

ISBN 978–1–84709–104–8

1 3 5 7 9 10 8 6 4 2

Typeset by Fakenham Photosetting Ltd, Fakenham, Norfolk
Printed in Great Britain by Ashford Colour Press

Produced on paper from sustainable forests

# Contents

# Preface

Who would want to read a book on prostate cancer? At first thought, very few. If you already know you have it, or your partner or a close relative has it, you are an obvious potential reader. If you think you might be developing it, you are another. If you have the odd problem with your ability to urinate, maybe struggling to maintain your flow or being unable to get it started easily, you may be wondering about your prostate health.

This book aims to help you all, but it is also for a much wider readership. It is for anyone with an interest in enjoying a healthy old age, regardless of whether or not you fear prostate cancer in particular. There are several reasons for this. Most important among them is the fact that prostate cancer is almost the 'hidden epidemic' among us. While breast, lung and bowel cancers hit the headlines time and again when a new treatment for them is launched, the constant stream of good news about prostate cancer coming from the research institutes and hospitals never seems to excite the editors.

Partly that is because most of us know little about the prostate gland and its importance. That goes as much for the media people who write and broadcast about health matters as for their readers, listeners and viewers. Even the most prestigious newspaper, magazine, radio and television journalists still persist in misspelling and misstating 'prostate' as 'prostrate'! I have had my own written copy for health columns miscorrected in this way many times by subeditors: it makes me frustrated and angry. If people whose very job depends on their excellent knowledge of the English language get such things wrong, there is little chance that you are as well informed as you should be.

That is sad, because in countries where huge efforts have been made to educate the public about prostate cancer, deaths from the disease have passed their peak and may even be declining. The hidden epidemic is no longer hidden in the USA. Better public awareness of prostate cancer there has led to earlier diagnosis and therefore to earlier and more successful treatment. Combine these pieces of good news with newer treatments that cure or give long-term relief from prostate cancers, and the war against them is beginning to be won. The American Cancer Society, using figures from the US National Cancer Institute, has shown that since the early 1990s deaths from prostate cancer have been declining each year – the total fall is now around 10 per cent.

This welcome fall in deaths from prostate cancer is not because there have been fewer cases. On the contrary, prostate cancer cases have been rising all over the developed world, the USA included. The rise is expected to continue and become steeper as more men in each country reach old age. In 1994, Drs R. and M. Kirby and Drs J. and A. Fitzpatrick predicted the increase in numbers of men over 60 years old in various countries by the year 2020. The projected increase for the UK was the lowest, at 60 per cent. The figures for the USA, Japan and Canada were 120, 160 and 210 per cent, respectively. Writing now in 2010, I can say that they were an underestimate.

Why are these figures relevant to prostate cancer? Our risk of developing it, more than for any other cancer, rises steeply as we age. That doesn't mean that everyone with prostate cancer is so old that there's not much point in treating them. Far from it. The rise in risk starts at ages 50–54, with 8 in every 1000 men of that age developing prostate cancer. The figure rises to:

- 23 in every 1000 men by ages 55–59;
- 68 in every 1000 men by ages 60–64;
- 140 in every 1000 men by ages 65–69; and
- 260 in every 1000 men by ages 70–74.

Prostate cancer is number three in the causes of early death from cancer, after breast cancer in women and lung cancer in both sexes.

So my aim in writing this book is to help to reduce these figures. The best way to do this is to persuade more men to seek early diagnosis of any small symptoms related to passing urine. Only a few turn out to be due to prostate cancer, but it is vital to sort them out from all the other, more minor causes. That is because the earlier your prostate cancer is diagnosed, the better chance you have of complete cure. Today, around half of all prostate cancers have already spread outside the boundaries of the gland at the time of diagnosis; at this stage they cannot be completely removed. I describe in this book the many new treatments for this stage of cancer that prolong life and ease the symptoms, but it can't yet be completely cured. We are constantly striving to initiate ways of catching far more prostate cancers earlier, when they are curable. As most of them grow slowly and predictably, an early diagnosis makes cure more feasible than for other cancers.

There is one group of men whose prostate cancers can be diagnosed at an earlier stage still, when they have no symptoms at all. Heredity can play a big part. If your father, brother, or uncle has had the disease at a younger age than most, say in their 50s, you could be at higher than normal risk. If you can go back further in your family tree you may find more men who have died early from the disease. This is a very good reason for you to be 'screened' for prostate disease. Tests for detecting the earliest stages of prostate cancer are improving rapidly, and a chapter of this book has been devoted to them.

Should we apply such screening for early prostate cancer to the general population? In the first edition of this book, written in 2001, the idea was being promoted in the press and by some experts. Today, in 2010, with much more evidence for and against the techniques used in screening, we have become a little less enthusiastic. I've updated the chapter on screening and diagnosis accordingly, giving the pros and cons of screening. I leave you to decide for yourself which aspect of the medical arguments that are currently raging in the medical journals apply to you. That's not a cop-out. Everyone is different, and what applies to one man may not necessarily apply to another.

The big question is what do we do about screening for the disease in men with no history of the disease in the family and no symptoms of early prostate cancer? Many small prostate cancers found on screening will never progress in the man's expected lifetime to a stage where they will cause symptoms, far less death, from the disease itself. Finding them would be a disadvantage, as it would add unnecessary stress and fear to the man's life. So the section of this book that deals with screening also looks at how to separate the prostate cancers that are likely to progress and become life-threatening from those that can be left alone. We are still not very good at making this vital distinction, but we are improving.

The first part of this book is therefore about diagnosis of prostate cancer. It is for men who have heard of it and would like to know more about it – so it should interest all men in middle age and beyond. The second part is about its treatment. It is for men, and their concerned partners, relatives and friends, who have had to face the diagnosis.

Now for the good news. Even in the second decade of the twenty-first century, people often link the word 'cancer' with imminent death. The book's section on treatment firmly dispels that view. The people who are waging the war on prostate cancer are universally optimistic about winning it. Surgeons have found better ways to remove diseased prostate glands, while preserving sexual function and sensation (a real drawback in the past). Physicians have found better drugs and other methods to slow and even arrest the spread of the disease. More optimistically still, as we learn much more about the ways in which prostate cancers start and then spread within the body, the molecular biologists and geneticists are co-ordinating and combining their knowledge to develop ways of reversing the disease. Their results are already reaching cancer clinics, and are producing results.

My overall message is that:

Men with prostate cancer can live successfully, happily and with fulfilment. This is the book's overall message. If you or a partner, relative or friend have the illness, please read it. It aims to support and lighten the burden, and not to depress.

Here I must pay a debt to several doctors without whom this book could not have been written. First to Dr Jonathan Waxman, of London, with whom I worked some years ago. He guided me and first fired my special interest in this disease. Then to two other Londoners, Roger Kirby and Timothy Christmas, and their colleague Michael Brawer, of Seattle. Together these three men wrote the definitive book for doctors on prostate cancer (*Prostate Cancer*, 2nd edition, published by Elsevier, 2001). As a GP, I obviously do not have their personal experience of research and of the specialist treatments in which they are so expert. So in the first, 2001, edition of this book I drew on their book for many of my facts. Any reader, medical or not, who would like to know much more about prostate disease could not do better than read their book. It is beautifully written and illustrated, though it will hardly be used as a coffee table ornament! Since 2001, I have drawn on the progress reported in the medical journals to keep the book up to date.

My thanks, too, go to my editor, Fiona Marshall, of Sheldon Press, for her invaluable advice on style and content. Medicine is not the only discipline that changes with the years – literature develops too. I hope that my changes in style and format make this new edition easier to read.

*Note*: This is not a medical book and is not intended to replace advice from your doctor. Do consult your doctor if you are experiencing symptoms with which you feel you need help.

# 1

# The normal prostate gland

Let's first make the name clear. It is the 'prostate' gland, not the 'prostrate' gland. Prostrate things lie flat – that's nothing to do with prostate, which is derived from the ancient Greek, meaning 'to stand in front of'. The word was first applied to what we now know as the prostate gland, according to medical historians, by Herophilus, a Greek living in Alexandria around 335 BC. Herophilus was slightly out in his anatomy, because it lies beneath, rather than in front of the bladder. He can be forgiven for that small mistake, because doctors did not add to his knowledge of the gland in the following 2000 years.

## Structure and functions of the prostate

Why do we have a prostate gland? It provides most of the fluid that forms the ejaculate. The testes provide the sperm, which passes along tubes upwards through the groin and into the abdomen, where they collect in the seminal vesicles, small 'bags' lying just above the prostate. During ejaculation, sperm from the seminal vesicles mixes with a much larger volume of fluid from the prostate gland to form the ejaculate, or semen.

To function normally, therefore, the prostate must be made up of two main tissues:

- the glands and ducts that form and transport the fluid; and
- muscle fibres that provide the power to propel the fluid out of the prostate into the urethra – the tube from bladder to penis through which the ejaculate must flow during orgasm.

The prostate is therefore wrapped around the base of the bladder,

1

rectum

bladder

seminal
vesicle

prostate

anus

thigh

urethra

**Figure 1.1 The prostate gland and its relationships to the bladder
and nerve plexus.**

surrounding the urethra. It is the size and consistency of a small
orange (such as a tangerine), with the two seminal vesicles lying
above and to the side of it. The ducts within the prostate lead
into an opening in the urethra (Figure 1). Above the prostate lies
the base of the bladder, within the walls of which are muscle
and nerve fibres that are very sensitive to the pressure of urine
within the bladder. Also around the side of the prostate is the
network (the medical word is 'plexus') of nerves that control
and co-ordinate the outflow of urine from the bladder as well as
erection and ejaculation.

## What happens when the prostate enlarges

Bear these anatomical facts in mind when trying to understand
why problems with the prostate produce such diverse symptoms. For example, when the prostate enlarges for any reason, it
can compress the urethra. Naturally that makes it more difficult

to pass urine. Because the urine is passing through a narrower tube, you need more force to expel it, and the flow can be slower and more difficult to sustain or maintain.

If disease of the prostate invades upwards, it can put pressure on the base of the bladder. That can upset bladder control, so that you may feel you need to pass urine more often than normal ('frequency'), or the signal of needing to pass urine may be stronger and more pressing than normal ('urgency'), or you may get feelings of incomplete emptying of the bladder.

Invading in other directions, disease of the prostate may interfere with the nerve plexus around it, causing impotence, or interfering with ejaculation. It may destroy sexual feelings in the penis. And disease within the prostate can cause internal bleeding in the organ so that blood appears in the ejaculated sperm.

Of course, there are other causes of all these symptoms (such as a bladder infection or an infection in the prostate – 'prostatitis') than cancer, but any one of them should alert you to the possibility that they may be due to it.

## The zones of the prostate

To understand what can go wrong with the prostate it's good to know a little about its structure. We divide it into three zones. Figure 2 shows how these three zones all relate to each other and to the urethra, the seminal vesicles and the base of the bladder.

The lower two-thirds of the prostate – the part that doctors can reach with their fingers from the anus – is where most cancers start. That's why we look on rectal examination as so important, despite you sometimes finding it a little distasteful and uncomfortable.

Most of the upper third of the gland is taken up with what we call the 'central' zone, which lies just underneath the bladder and behind the urethra. If it enlarges, it can narrow the urethra and irritate the base of the bladder.

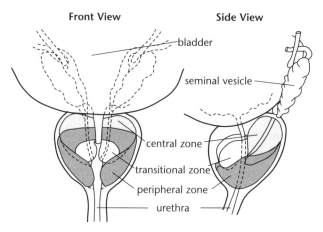

**Figure 2** **The three zones of the prostate and how they relate to rectal examination.**

Between 5 and 10 per cent of the prostate consists of the 'transition' zone, which wraps around the upper third of the urethra, in front of the central zone. Most cases of benign enlargement of the prostate arise in this zone, so that it usually causes bladder and urethral symptoms (the frequency, urgency, and poor flow) earlier than does prostate cancer, which needs to enlarge far more than benign tumours in the transition zone do to cause problems.

The medical term for benign prostate enlargement is benign prostatic hyperplasia (BPH), also sometimes called benign prostatic hypertrophy. It is by far the main cause of prostate symptoms, and is far more common than prostate cancer. A skilled doctor can usually tell the difference between the two, at least when the diseases are in their early stages.

It is also important to understand that all cells in the prostate, regardless of the zone they are in, produce substances called prostate-specific antigen (PSA) and prostatic acid phosphatase (PAP), about which much more is explained later in this book. They are important in diagnosing and following the progression of prostate cancer. Two more substances crucial to understanding prostate cancer are growth factors and androgens. It is enough to state here that growth factors seem to be more concentrated in the central and transition zones and androgen receptors in the peripheral zones. Knowing about this has led researchers to a new understanding of ways to combat prostate cancer.

As mentioned above, most prostate cancers (more than 70 per cent) arise in the lower two-thirds of the gland, making them relatively easy to feel with a finger in the anus. Unfortunately such cancers arise near the neural plexus that controls the blood flow to the penis. That makes them more likely to cause early sexual problems, such as impotence and failure of ejaculation. The next chapter describes in greater detail how an enlarging prostate can cause problems.

# 2

# When the prostate goes wrong – the natural history of prostate cancer

## Finding the cancers that may kill

Most men with recognized prostate cancer are beyond their middle age: they are over 70. Many such cancers progress very slowly, so that if you are given the diagnosis at this age, you can live 10 years or more with your disease, eventually dying from a quite unconnected problem, such as a heart attack or stroke. This has led to some doctors suggesting that most prostate cancers are better not found, because they only cause us to worry unnecessarily about dying from a disease that is ultimately not going to kill us.

There is good reason for this viewpoint. There are small areas of cancer in the prostates of one in five men who have died from other causes in their 20s, in one in three men dying in their 50s, and in seven in every ten men over 80 – microscopic areas of cancer that had caused no symptoms in the men's lifetimes. If the men had survived the disease, or avoided the accident or even act of murder, that had killed them, very few of those cancers would eventually have developed enough to become obvious. The vast majority develop very slowly, if at all. A more realistic assessment of your risk is that fewer than one in ten men develop symptoms of prostate cancer in their lifetime, and fewer than three in 100 die from the disease.

So we really need to detect early those cancers that do go on to develop, that somehow escape the body's mechanisms that protect us against them. Happily, we are getting much better at doing just that.

## Inheriting prostate cancer

The first pointer to better protection against progressive prostate cancer is that if you have had a relative with the disease you have a higher than expected chance of developing it than if your family is clear of it. In a 1960 study, the fathers and brothers of men with prostate cancer were three times more likely to have the disease than those of men without it. Among Mormons in the USA, prostate cancer had a stronger tendency to be inherited than bowel or breast cancer. Men with two close relatives with prostate cancer had five times the lifetime risk of the illness than people with no such relatives, and men with three close relatives with it had 11 times the risk. One in 11 prostate cancers has a genetic background.

This news has two consequences. One is that all men with prostate cancer in the family should be regularly screened for the earliest signs of the disease. This should start at a relatively young age, say around 40 years, because inherited prostate cancers usually show themselves much earlier in life and are more aggressive in their behaviour than those in men with no relatives with the disease. If we can detect them early, before they produce symptoms, today's surgical and medical methods offer a near 100 per cent chance of cure.

So far the exact site or sites of the problem genes have not been identified, but we think that the change that leads to the cancer involves loss of, or mutation in, a gene that normally suppresses cancerous change, and that this gene lies either on chromosome 1 (of our 23 pairs of genes) or on the X chromosome. This is no place for a detailed description of how genetics can be manipulated to help to cure cancers, but this information does offer hope, in that researchers are on the way towards finding practical methods of restoring defective genes to normal.

## Geography makes a difference

Another clue to the origins of prostate cancer is the wide varia-
tion between countries in their incidence of the disease. The
Scandinavians have the highest prostate cancer detection rates,
at around 60 cases per 100,000 men per year. This compares
with figures of 50 in the USA, 20 in the UK, and only four in
China and Japan. Why should these figures be so different? The
numbers of deaths from prostate cancer in the USA and the UK
do not differ nearly so much – they are 20 per hundred thousand in America and 12 per hundred thousand in the UK. These
figures strongly suggest that many men diagnosed as having
early prostate cancer in the USA (who are exposed to strong
pressures to be 'screened') would not develop obvious disease
if left without treatment, and might be better left undiagnosed.

However, earlier diagnosis from better screening alone does
not explain why Japanese emigrating to California or Hawaii
have more than twice the prostate cancer rate of those living
in Japan (though still far less prostate cancer than Californians
of European or African descent or native Hawaiians). There are
similar rising figures for migrants into the USA from China and
India. The common theme running through all these studies is
that there is a basic incidence of prostate cancer in every com-
munity that may be increased by some environmental factors,
the main one probably being diet. But there are other factors,
such as levels of male sex hormones, that must be taken into
consideration.

## Male sex hormones

The prostate gland cannot develop to maturity without male sex
hormones circulating in the blood. They are collectively known
as androgens, the best known of which is testosterone. So the
prostate gland remains small until puberty, when we become
awash with testosterone. Along with acne and our awakening

interest in the opposite sex come a rapidly enlarging and functioning prostate gland.

However, testosterone has its drawbacks, one of which is that prostate cancer only develops if we are producing it. Without testosterone, no one gets prostate cancer. Men who inherit deficits in sex hormone production – medically speaking they are 'pseudohermaphrodites' – do not develop mature prostate glands, or prostate cancer. Nor do eunuchs. However, there is no direct relationship between the levels of testosterone in our bloodstream and our risk of prostate cancer. It is not true that the higher our testosterone level, the greater the risk we have of developing prostate cancer. In fact, it is only as we grow older, and our testosterone levels are falling with age, that the cancers start to show themselves.

One reason for this is the long latent period between the first cancerous change in a prostate cell and the cancers becoming big enough to give symptoms. Another is the fact that testosterone is not the real culprit. Inside the prostate gland, testosterone is converted into a much more active hormone, dihydrotestosterone, or DHT, by the enzyme 5-alpha-reductase. This may seem a bit too technical for a book like this, but it is important to know about it, because this reaction is the basis for one of the most successful means of treating prostate cancer. DHT, and not testosterone, is now known to be the androgen that stimulates the growth of the prostate in puberty, and it is DHT that is needed to keep the mature prostate working at maximum efficiency during men's sexual lives. Its downside is that it is also a powerful stimulus to prostate cancer cells to keep growing.

That is one of the many areas of new knowledge about prostate cancer in the past 30 years that offers hope for its treatment. Once researchers knew about 5-alpha-reductase and its activity in producing DHT, they were soon working on drugs to block its action, and so stop the growth of prostate cancer cells. There is now a series of drugs for prostate cancer, the 5-alpha-reductase inhibitors, that do exactly that. They are widely used not just to shrink tumours in the prostate gland itself but also to reduce the volume of 'metastases', secondary areas of prostate cancer distant from the initial (or 'primary') site.

Evidence that 5-alpha-reductase is important in prostate cancer comes from studies of men who are born without the ability to produce it. They form one group of the pseudo-hermaphrodite men mentioned above: their prostate glands remain in the pre-pubertal state, and never become cancerous. Differences in inherited levels of 5-alpha-reductase may also explain, at least partly, the big variations in prostate cancer rates in different areas of the world. A 1992 report in the *Lancet* proposed that the lower prostate cancer rate in Japan is linked to the fact that Japanese men have, on average, much lower levels of 5-alpha-reductase than men elsewhere.

We have known for many years, too, that men with cirrhosis of the liver are much less likely than normal to develop prostate cancer. This has been linked to the finding that cirrhosis leads to lower levels of testosterone, and higher levels of the female sex hormone oestrogen, than is normal in men. Both of these hormonal changes in theory should reduce any risk of developing prostate cancer.

## What you eat and prostate cancer

Oestrogens are present in food, so some foods should also protect against prostate cancer. One reason behind the low incidence of prostate cancer in Japanese and Chinese men is that they eat many more root and green vegetables than men in the West. Present in such vegetables, particularly in soya, are plant-based oestrogens (phyto-oestrogens) called genistein and daidzein. Men who eat enough of them alter the balance of male and female sex hormones in their blood – and that change is enough to lower their risk of prostate cancer. Japanese men who have taken to Western eating habits and eat fewer vegetables have a higher rate of prostate cancer than those who stick to their own style of eating.

Phyto-oestrogens are not the only substances in food that may influence our chances of developing prostate cancer. The high numbers of cases in the USA have been linked to the eating of high amounts of animal fats mainly derived from dairy products and red meats. In the USA, the regions in which people eat the most fats and dairy products are also those with the highest prostate cancer rates. In a strict follow-up over many years of 4700 men working in the health professions (the US Health Professionals Study), 300 developed prostate cancer. They had eaten significantly more red meat than the others who had no prostate disease. The link was strongest among Asian Americans.

Why should eating fats increase prostate cancer risk? One possible cause, taken from animal studies, suggests that fats speed up the change from normal cells to cancer cells in a prostate influenced by testosterone levels. Another is that eating high amounts of animal fats reduces our ability to absorb vitamin A. This reduces the blood levels of beta-carotene, the active form of the vitamin, which is thought to help to prevent prostate cancer from developing. Vegetables are high in vitamin A, and when men change to a vegetarian, low-fat diet their blood testosterone levels fall by 30 per cent. This should also lower the chance of testosterone-stimulated prostate cancer.

On the whole, therefore, if you eat mainly foods high in animal fats and eat few vegetables you must face the fact that you are raising your risk of prostate cancer.

It isn't good, either, to try to change your diet simply by taking vitamin or mineral supplements. Your answer is, rather, to eat better. The addition of vitamin E (alpha-tocopherol) or vitamin A (beta-carotene) to the normal eating patterns of men produced mixed, even startling, results. Vitamin E supplements, for example, were reported to reduce prostate cancer rates, but only in smokers, yet prostate cancer is one of the few cancers not definitively linked to smoking. Beta-carotene supplements have actually been linked to increases in prostate cancer in two separate studies, one in the USA ( Heinonen *et al.*, *Journal of the National Cancer Institute*, 1998, volume 90, pages 440–6), and one in Scandinavia (Tretli *et al.*, *Journal of the National Cancer Institute*, 1996, volume 88, page 128).

## Possible effects of sunshine and vitamin D

There is even research to suggest that prostate cancer cases increase the further we live from the equator, possibly because at higher latitudes we have less vitamin D in our tissues. Vitamin D levels are lower, generally, in people who are exposed to less overhead sunshine. The skin makes the vitamin from sunlight. In the laboratory, adding vitamin D to cultures of prostate cancer cells prevents them from becoming cancerous and multiplying out of control, but studies of populations with different vitamin D levels in their blood have not confirmed that higher levels of it prevent prostate cancer onset or spread.

## No link with sexual activity?

Because the prostate's only function is to produce the right quantity and quality of seminal fluid, it has been assumed that prostate cancer may be linked to excessive sexual activity. It was proposed that, compared with average, men who start sex early, who have multiple sexual partners, who may have had sexually transmitted diseases, and who have more frequent sex over more years are at higher risk of the disease. That is difficult to judge because we have too little information from enough men to know what is the norm and how many differ from it.

The results of studies on the subjects only confuse us further. One study proposed a link between prostate cancer and gonorrhoea caught around 45 years earlier; another study suggested a relationship between lower than normal sexual activity in men and increases in prostate cancer rates. The bravest study looked at deaths from prostate cancer in 1400 Roman Catholic priests. We have to assume that, being avowedly celibate, they had had much less sexual experience than the rest of the male population! They had just the same death rate from prostate cancer as other men.

So we can't draw any conclusions on whether sexual activity increases or decreases the risk of prostate cancer, or whether it makes no difference. If having sex earlier and having more sexual partners do indeed make a difference to prostate cancer rates, then we will find out soon, because in the past 30 years the average age at first intercourse for British men has dropped from 20 years to 17 years, and the average number of sexual partners that men have in a lifetime has increased steeply over the same time. By, say, 2030, we may be recording steep rises in prostate cancer cases.

## Other influences on prostate cancer

### Pollutants

In 1994, Chinese doctors reported that prostate cancers were more common in cities than in country districts, and that city men were more likely than country men to die from them. They suggested that industrial pollution might provoke prostate cancer. They listed workers exposed to chemicals in the rubber, textile, chemicals, drugs, fertilizer, and atomic energy industries as being at high risk of prostate cancer. Which chemicals may be the direct cause they did not know, but one chemical high on the suspect list is cadmium. The atomic energy industry in Britain has been seeking connections between prostate cancer and radioactive forms of hydrogen, chromium, iron, cobalt and zinc. So far, none has been proved.

## Viruses

Could prostate cancer be the result of a viral infection? Viruses are known to 'trigger' the development of other cancers, including cervical cancer in women, so it is feasible for viruses to do the same in men. The difficulty has been in identifying possible virus candidates from prostate cancer material. A typical study reported antibodies to herpes simplex virus type 2 (well known to the public as 'genital herpes', and linked to cervical cancer in women) in the blood of 71 per cent of men with prostate cancer and 66 per cent of men with BPH. The detection in blood of antibodies to a virus indicates a past infection with the virus. Herpes virus has been detected in prostate cancer cells, and one study, not yet confirmed by others, suggested that wives of men with prostate cancer are at higher than usual risk of cancer of the cervix.

For the moment, the jury is out on whether viruses may cause prostate cancer. If eventually they are found to do so, this leaves the way open to exciting new treatments: but antiviral drugs for prostate cancer are still a long way off. I wrote about this first in 2004: sadly, in 2010, there is still no prospect of them.

## Vasectomy

Probably the most contentious issue surrounding prostate cancer is whether or not it may be caused by a previous vasectomy, perhaps many years before. The proposal that the operation may lead to cancerous change in the prostate was raised in 1990, and seemed to be confirmed by two more studies in 1993, but eventually much larger studies (published in 1999) failed to find a link. More than 10 years later, there have been no further claims that vasectomy can cause prostate cancer changes.

These conflicting results leave doctors like myself in a quandary. Many couples ask for advice on vasectomy. It is widely held to be safe and harmless. The evidence suggests that there may be a very small risk that it may cause prostate cancer in a few men. Or there may be none at all. I used to tell men considering vasectomy that a future small risk of prostate cancer is a possibility, but now I'm more positive about the operation. If you have had no close relative with prostate cancer, I explain that you are either at very low or no extra risk of getting it yourself. You then discuss it with your partner, and usually you will go ahead with the vasectomy. On the other hand, if you are already at higher risk (because of a father or brother with the disease), I tend to advise against vasectomy, for two reasons. One is that we do not know for certain if vasectomy might give you an added risk, on top of your already higher than average one, so it seems foolish to take the chance. The second reason is that if you eventually develop prostate cancer after a vasectomy, you will feel guilty and blame yourself, even if it is not the cause, for submitting to the operation. That is no mental attitude with which to fight the disease.

## BPH and prostate cancer – are they related?

If you already have BPH (benign prostatic hyperplasia), it is natural to ask whether your BPH will turn into prostate cancer. Here, as with vasectomy, the researchers have come to different conclusions. At first sight, a link between the two is unlikely: the two diseases arise mostly in two different zones of the prostate – cancer in the peripheral zone, BPH in the transition zone. In 1974, however, two prestigious medical journals reported diametrically opposite studies on this question. Armenian and colleagues reported in the *Lancet* that men with BPH subsequently develop prostate cancer three times more often than men with apparently normal prostate glands. Greenwald and colleagues, reporting in the *Journal of the National Cancer Institute*, found a reduced risk of prostate cancer in men with BPH.

What is the poor GP to think of that?

The fact is that both BPH and prostate cancer are common in older men, so that by chance it is likely that both diseases will co-exist in many men, without the first having developed into the second. I see no need to add to the existing worries of men with BPH by suggesting that they need extra tests to rule out cancer, or that they must be extra vigilant because they are at higher than normal risk of developing it. The evidence suggests that they are not.

## How the cancer will progress – if it does

So you have just been told you have prostate cancer. Your next question is, obviously, what is going to happen to me? How is it going to develop? Am I going to die soon? Usually we can be very positive and optimistic in answering you. Today's treatments are very successful. Surgery, radiotherapy, cryotherapy (freezing) and drug treatments all alter the course of the disease and may eradicate it altogether. But what about leaving the cancer alone, and letting it follow its natural course?

That sounds stupid and cruel – but it may not be. Consider the fact that in 1994 Dr G. W. Chodak and colleagues collected and analysed the results of letting the disease take its natural course, with no medical or surgical intervention, in 828 men whose prostate cancers were confined to the gland itself (Chodak *et al.*, *New England Journal of Medicine*, 1994, volume 330, pages 242–8). It would be impossible to repeat their research today, because there is too much pressure on doctors to treat every prostate cancer actively, with surgery, radiotherapy or medical treatment. Yet many doctors like myself wonder, after the Chodak group's results, whether some men with prostate cancer would not be far better untreated.

The Chodak report showed that 94 per cent of the men whose cancers were, on the basis of their microscopic appearance, well differentiated survived for at least 10 years after their diagnosis.

This was in contrast to only 58 per cent of the men whose tumours were classified as poorly differentiated. A 94 per cent survival in men of their age is virtually normal, so it is reasonable to conclude that treating these men would not have offered them any advantage over just 'waiting and seeing' how they got on.

The crucial point about the Chodak findings is the phrase 'well differentiated'. This means that the cancer cells seen under the microscope still look like prostate cells. They are clearly cancerous, but they are not the fast-multiplying 'undifferentiated' cells that will produce a rapidly growing tumour. They may be so slow growing that they will never enlarge enough to cause pressure on the bladder, the urethra and the nerve plexus around the prostate or to invade into the blood vessels around it. In effect, if you have this type of tumour you will probably never have serious problems with it. You may be one of the men who have such tumours in their 20s – tumours that have never developed beyond the microscopic state.

The poorly differentiated tumour is different in outlook. Its cells look much less like their parent normal prostate cells. Instead they are a mass of cells with no obvious normal prostate tissue among them. They have much denser centres: in a single 'field' under the microscope there will be several cells that are obviously dividing – splitting into daughter cells. They are the cancers that will spread, form obvious masses within the prostate and outside it, and eventually lead to early death. They must be treated aggressively with all that the cancer team can throw at them.

This knowledge leaves doctors in a dilemma. The decision to deal with the poorly differentiated type of cancer is easy to take – it has to be treated and eradicated if possible. But what should be done about the well-differentiated types? A small minority of them will become more aggressive if left to themselves. The problem is how to predict which will do so. The various tests in which 'prostate markers' are used to try to do this are explained later, but they are not perfectly reliable. So in practice, everyone with a diagnosis of prostate cancer is now treated, so as to ensure that those that will change to a more malignant phase will be dealt with.

## The stages of prostate cancer

There are three main steps in the development of aggressive prostate cancer:

- The earliest phase is the appearance of microscopic clusters of cancer cells within the prostate gland, which produce no symptoms and cannot be detected by normal physical examination.
- The second phase is when these cells start to grow in bulk within the prostate gland to a size that is detectable by physical examination and is starting to cause symptoms, such as urinary problems.
- The third phase is when the cancer spreads outside the prostate gland into the tissues immediately surrounding it, such as lymph glands in the pelvis and abdomen, and then distantly into bones, such as spinal vertebrae.

How this progression occurs is still a matter of fairly heated argument among the experts. Some doctors believe that all prostate cancers eventually follow this route from stage one to stage three in time and that some are simply slower than others in doing so. It has been shown that it can take four years for a prostate cancer to double in size, so that it may be ten years before it reaches one millilitre in volume. This is the size at which many cancers start to cause symptoms, although many more are undetected until they are two or three times as big as this.

Other researchers propose that for prostate cancers to progress they need to undergo several successive genetic mutations. The first mutation may produce the well-differentiated cancers mentioned above, but they need a second mutation to turn them into aggressive undifferentiated cancers, and perhaps a third to cause them to spread further than the prostate. The chances of men having three successive mutations in a cancer are very small, which is why aggressive, life-threatening cancers are relatively rare. This could be why so many men with microscopic cancers never go on to have serious disease.

This 'multistep' explanation for the development of cancer may also explain why, although microscopic prostate cancer rates are similar all over the world, the rates of aggressive, spreading cancers differ widely. In the countries with the higher prostate cancer death rates, environmental conditions that lead to mutations may be changing the nature of the disease.

How these mutations can happen is explained in more detail in the next chapter. By necessity it is complex, so that you can skip it, and turn to Chapters 4 and 5, which describe the ways in which prostate cancers show themselves. However, if you wish to know the latest thinking on how prostate cancer arises and develops further, then Chapter 3 is a must for you.

# 3

# The science behind prostate cancer

The prostate gland has a very complex architecture. Its cells produce fluid of very intensely controlled composition within closely defined limits for maximum benefit for the sperm. The prostate contains:

- ducts (channels) that collect the fluid;
- muscle cells that expel the fluid from the ducts;
- fibres that supply the 'skeleton' for the gland;
- nerves to co-ordinate the function of all these elements; and
- blood vessels to supply oxygen and nutrients.

None of these structures is static. The cells within them are constantly dying off and being renewed. They are continually exposed to the effects of hormones and growth factors that stimulate their growth, and to the effects of genes that initiate their 'suicide' when they are too old to function normally or are showing signs of becoming cancerous. It is when the balance between growth and death of cells is disturbed that prostate cancers start. This brief chapter summarizes the latest thoughts and knowledge about how that disturbance can occur.

## The effects of male sex hormones

The foremost influence on prostate cell growth is the male sex hormones. The best known of these to the public is testosterone. It is popularly a synonym for male strength and sexual potency. Testosterone itself is made in the testes, and, as mentioned earlier, without it the prostate cannot develop. However, the testes are not the only source of male sex hormone. A small amount (much less than formed in the testes) is made by the adrenal glands, which lie over the upper surface of the kidneys. They produce two 'androgens' – hormones like testosterone that stimulate male sexual function – called androstene and androstenedione.

In normal circumstances, the effect of adrenal androgens on the prostate is tiny, as they are overwhelmed by the effects of testosterone. But if all testosterone is removed, such as by castration, or by drugs that block the effect of testosterone, then the adrenal androgens will still continue to stimulate prostate growth. This effect is vital when it comes to treating prostate cancer – it is sometimes necessary to remove the effect of adrenal, as well as testicular, male sex hormone from the prostate cancer cells. How this is done is explained in more detail in Chapter 15.

## The role of 5-alpha-reductase

The effects of testosterone and adrenal androgens on the prostate are not straightforward. To stimulate prostate cell growth they must first be converted, within the prostate, into dihydrotestosterone (DHT). This is done by a substance also produced in the prostate, called 5-alpha-reductase. If the action of 5-alpha-reductase can be blocked, then the prostate cells, whether normal or cancerous, lose the biggest stimulus to their growth. Without 5-alpha-reductase, the cell suicide pathway is unopposed. Within ten days of starting treatment to block 5-alpha-reductase, 90 per cent of the prostate cells undergo suicide.

This is why one of the first attacks on prostate cancer, or, for that matter, benign prostatic overgrowth or BPH for many men is a drug to block 5-alpha-reductase. But it is not the only chink in the prostate cancer cell armoury.

## Genetic effects on prostate cells

New genetic techniques have identified genes in the prostate that stimulate the cell suicide process. Genes are usually given a three-letter identity and sometimes a number, and convention dictates they are printed in italics. The 'good' genes, as far as prostate cancer is concerned, in that they promote cancer cell suicide, are *bax* and *bcl-2*. Another family of genes needed for control of normal cell growth is called *Cdc2*. They work along with a protein called cyclin to help prostate cells grow in an orderly, non-cancerous fashion.

### Growth factors

Genes exert these effects by forming substances called growth factors. There's no need here to explain how growth factors stimulate cells to grow and multiply: it is enough that growth factors have been identified in prostate tissue. They include epidermal growth factor, insulin-like growth factor, fibroblast growth factor and transforming growth factor, among several others. Named mainly after the tissue or system that they stimulate, they are vital in our plans for future treatments of prostate cancer. If the growth factor that stimulates the growth of a particular cancer can be identified and its effects neutralized, or if it can be destroyed, then that cancer will stop growing. Trials of drugs that block specific growth factors are, as I write in 2010, under way.

## Mechanism of cancer growth

So how do prostate cancers start, and then continue? Knowledge of hormones, genes and growth factors has given us many clues. Cancer of any tissue starts when a mutation, or several mutations, occur inside a cell that gives it an advantage in growth (or in resisting the message to commit suicide) over the cells surrounding it. No longer responding to the normal controls, it starts to produce daughter cells by dividing in two. (Cells divide in order to multiply, a curious anomaly for the mathematical mind.) As the numbers of its descendants increase, there is an increasing chance that one of them will undergo a further mutation, and the cancer will become less like the original normal cell. In medical terms, it becomes de-differentiated. This process eventually leads to the cells developing an ability to spread through the surface of the prostate to the surrounding tissues in the pelvis, and then, by breaking into blood vessels, being carried in the circulation to distant sites in the body, where they can lodge and grow. This is called metastasis.

This series of cancer-inducing steps takes time, which is why most prostate cancers do not make themselves obvious until later middle age or old age. But it is common in the longer run: the experts predict that around 9 per cent of all men develop prostate cancer in their lifetimes. Thankfully, only a small minority of this 9 per cent go on to die from their cancers.

## Stimulation of cell growth

Why do some men get them, and not others? For the answer we must go back to those genes. Some men possess oncogenes; that is, genes that with a single mutation can alter the balance between growth and suicide in prostate cells. Many have already been identified. They include genes labelled as *ras, sis, c-erb, c-myc, c-fos* and *c-jun*. When these genes go wrong, they constantly give the cells the signal to grow and multiply and to ignore the suicide call. However, the body has its own way of protecting itself against oncogenes. It also possesses anti-oncogenes or tumour suppressor genes that oppose the activity of the oncogenes.

For example, one anti-oncogene was found by Professor David Lane and his team at Dundee University in Scotland. Called *p53,* it stimulates cell suicide when it detects any abnormality inside a cell that may suggest a pre-cancerous change. If *p53* is absent or bears a mutation that stops this vital function, the person has a highly increased risk of cancer, including prostate cancer. One research group found changes in the *p53* gene in up to 80 per cent of prostate cancer specimens.

## Breaking through the capsule of the prostate

Stimulation of cell growth is only the first step. For the cancer to spread outside the prostate it needs also to be able to break through the surface, known as the capsule. For that to happen, other genetic mutations have to happen. The cancer cells have to lose the natural tendency of prostate cells to stick together inside the architecture of the organ. Cells normally stick together by means of cell-adhesion molecules, called E-cadherin. The gene that forms E-cadherin is on chromosome 16 (we have 23 pairs of chromosomes plus the sex chromosomes XX or XY). If that gene fails, then cells easily burst through the prostate capsule to spread within the pelvis.

Once outside the prostate, the cancer cells need to have a blood supply to stay alive. Amazingly, researchers know how these cells form their own new source of blood. They secrete substances (called angiogenesis factors) that stimulate the growth of new blood vessels around them, so that they can survive and grow elsewhere in the body. There is even an 'antimetastatic factor' identified on chromosome 17, produced by gene *nm23*, that acts against the angiogenesis factors. When that is lost, the cancer can spread beyond control.

## How this information helps us

All this new scientific information may seem frightening to anyone who has prostate cancer or is caring for someone with the disease. It is not meant to frighten, but to reassure, because the more we know about the mechanisms that cause cancer first to develop and then to spread within the pelvis and to distant sites in the body, the better we are able to fight it. Already this knowledge has led to the development of drugs to block 5-alpha-reductase. They have had spectacular results in the clinic. Our knowledge of genes and chromosomes is leading to the identification of oncogenes, so that men at high risk can be watched to ensure that even the earliest change can be caught and dealt with as soon as it arises. New ways have been developed of identifying prostate cancer markers – substances that signal changes in chemistry before tumours are large enough to cause symptoms. One marker, prostate-specific antigen (PSA), is already being used routinely to identify cancers and to follow progress of treatment. It has a chapter to itself in this book (Chapter 7).

Although gene therapy is a few years away yet, there is progress towards ways of blocking oncogenes, renewing failed anti-oncogenes and tumour suppressor genes, and improving our immune system responses to prostate cancer.

We are already using androgen suppressor drugs to slow down and even arrest prostate cancers. We are drawing ever closer to finding medicines that will suppress the other growth factors that stimulate cancer cell growth, and to blocking angiogenesis. So there is optimism in the air among prostate cancer researchers and specialists. I hope this book can spread similar optimism among men with the disease, too.

# 4

# Some case histories

*James – a case from 40 years ago*
My first case history comes from nearly 40 years ago, in the early 1970s. It is here only to show how much our treatment of prostate cancer has improved over the last few decades. Please don't let it frighten you, because it is not what happens today.

James was 62 when he went to his doctor for the first time. He had not the slightest suspicion that he had anything wrong with his prostate gland. His main problem was pain low down in the centre of his back. It was there all the time, a persistent ache that never left him. It didn't matter what he was doing, bore no relation to the time of day, often kept him awake at night, and was neither worsened nor relieved by opening his bowel or his bladder. He didn't look well, was rather thinner than his doctor remembered from a year or two before, and admitted to vague tiredness and general lack of energy. He was shocked, when his doctor weighed him, to find he had lost nearly ten kilograms (a stone and a half). He thought that he had lost a little, but not that much.

This combination of loss of weight and persistent pain sounded ominous to his doctor, who decided to subject him to a thorough physical examination, a series of blood tests and some X-rays. The diagnosis became apparent on the rectal examination. The doctor's finger came up against a firm, non-tender swelling in the lower part of the prostate, quite discrete from the rest of the gland, which was smoother and softer to the touch. He was immediately referred to the local urology clinic, where after a further internal examination he was put on the only treatment then available, the female hormone oestrogen.

James' pain and feeling of ill-health improved very quickly. He was less tired and was able to return to work. But he had severe side effects. He lost his sexual drive, his chest began to change shape, so that he had feminine breasts that became embarrassing to him, and he lost his facial hair. He no longer had to shave, but he did not look on this as an advantage. Instead, he felt he was no longer a man. These side effects were tolerable because he knew the alternative, worsening bone pain, was even worse. James survived eight years before the cancer symptoms 'broke through' the oestrogen therapy. He then rapidly worsened, and died.

### Ian – a more recent case

Now, in 2010, men like James can look forward to a much better quality of life on their treatment for prostate cancer. Take Ian, the second case history, as a comparison. His first visit to his doctor was in April 2001. He had been a successful, physically very active, farmer all his life, and still walked over his fields and hill every day to check the stock. So when he started to feel a bit breathless and tired after only half a day's stroll, he thought something must be wrong. His only other symptoms were a persistent headache that did not respond easily to aspirin, and a difficulty in moving his right hip. He could not flex it up against his abdomen as easily as he could move his left thigh. His doctor confirmed that there was some restriction of movement of his right thigh but not of his left.

His doctor, who was also an old friend, was struck by his pale appearance and that he had lost some weight. So he took the symptoms seriously and arranged blood tests and an electrocardiogram (ECG). Ian turned out to be anaemic – his haemoglobin was around 12 grams, instead of the usual 15. There was nothing specific about the other blood tests, and his ECG was normal. But because he had not had a thorough check-up for some years, his doctor performed a rectal examination. The prostate was enlarged and had a firm, craggy 'feel', and it was larger on the right than on the left side. It seemed a bit 'stuck' against the surrounding tissues, and was not as easily moved about in the pelvis as a normal gland would be.

His doctor immediately sent him to the local hospital urological department, where the diagnosis of prostate cancer was confirmed. A test for prostate-specific antigen (PSA) was done, and a bone scan ordered. Happily, in that part of the UK, it was arranged within a week. The PSA turned out to be as high as 550 units, strongly suggestive that the cancer had spread beyond the confines of the prostate gland. Ian did not have to wait for treatment. It was started on the day he saw the consultant – a three-week course of cyproterone acetate pills, with an injection of goserelin acetate every three months (started a week after the first cyproterone pill). Within a few days he was feeling much better, and nine years later he is still in good health, though still on treatment. He understands that he will need it for the rest of his life. Without it he would have died, he knows, years ago.

Why Ian was given this treatment, the significance of the PSA test, and the need for the scan are explained in the next chapter (Chapter 5).

It suffices for the moment to use his case as an illustration of one way in which the illness is diagnosed.

Unfortunately, both Ian's case and James' case are, in reality, failures. Their prostate cancers were diagnosed too late for them to be cured, for their cancers to be eradicated altogether. Until around 1980, this was the way the vast majority of men found they had the disease. They came to their doctors only after they were losing weight, had pain in their bones, were tired all the time, had little energy and were having trouble passing or retaining urine. Treatments of advanced cancers like this have improved hugely over the years, but they still do not eradicate the disease completely. They often stave off death from prostate cancer until the men who have them die from something else, like a heart attack or stroke, or even 'old age', but the cancers remain in a relatively dormant state. There is always the possibility that they will become active and cause serious disease.

Happily, since the early 1980s we have become much better able to detect prostate cancers in their early stages, before they have spread, and that gives us the chance to remove them completely with new types of treatments and operations. The last half of this book is devoted to how we can do this now, and even improve in the future. So my third case history is about one of these more modern men, Frank.

### Frank

Frank's discovery that he might have prostate cancer came out of the blue. Called by his doctor for a 'well man' review on his 55th birthday, Frank was sure that he would be given a clean bill of health. He was fit and enjoying a successful life at the top of his career, and looking forward to some time with his wife now that the children were all grown and away from home.

One routine 'well man' test is a rectal examination. A finger gently inserted into the anus will detect abnormalities in the lower part of the bowel and the prostate. Frank did not find it uncomfortable or even unpleasant, but he was shocked to hear his doctor say that he might have a problem with his prostate. The finger had felt a small lump, harder than the rest of the prostate, near the lower surface of the gland.

His doctor explained that further blood tests would have to be performed, including a PSA test, and that he must see the local urologist, who had a special interest in prostate disease.

Events passed very quickly from then on. He saw the urologist that afternoon. He confirmed that it was probably a prostate cancer. The PSA measurement suggested that it was still localized to the gland itself, as did the ultrasound examination. For the first time in his life, Frank became concerned about his health. His doctors explained that there were two choices for him. One was to do nothing, and have repeated checks, every six months or so, of the size of the tumour, of the PSA level, and also of his general health. He was not anaemic and blood tests showed no problem with any other organs. A whole body scan to detect possible metastases was negative.

It came as a shock to Frank that he could have cancer yet his doctor could suggest that he might not need treatment. There was logic in this advice. Many prostate cancers are very slow growing and cause no problems for years. Treating them may be more of a bother to their 'owners' that waiting for them to become more active. That can take years.

One alternative for Frank was to remove the prostate gland in a 'radical prostatectomy', an operation that would remove the whole gland and with it the possibility of life-threatening disease. Another was to have radium seeds placed in his prostate gland, specifically arranged around the tumour to give a maximum chance of eradicating it. After a discussion with the consultant surgeon, and particularly because he was relatively young, Frank decided to go ahead with surgery. It was highly successful: Frank no longer needs to fear his prostate, and his PSA has dropped to the very minimum.

### Tony

In his 60s, Tony, like Frank, had his prostate cancer diagnosed by chance. His doctor had taken part in a trial to see if screening for cancer in the general population was worthwhile. Part of that screening was a routine PSA blood test. Tony's turned out to be well above normal – too high to ignore. Yet his prostate gland felt normal to the rectal examination. The ultrasound test showed no real change in the gland's make-up, and there was no obvious site from which a biopsy (removal of a piece of the gland for examination) could be taken. Tony's consultant was adamant about his management. He advised no treatment for the moment, and to take steps only if there was any change when Tony returned for follow-up over the next few months.

It wasn't easy for Tony to accept this policy of 'wait and see', but when it was explained that most prostate cancers were slow growing and any change would almost certainly be detected before it would threaten his life, he became reconciled to it. Now, eight years later, with no rise in his PSA and no obvious cancer developing, he is happy that he decided not to undergo surgery, with its discomfort and problems.

Tony's cancer was found on routine screening. Screening for prostate cancer in the general population is still controversial – unlike screening for breast cancer in women, which in 2001 was proved beyond all shadow of doubt to have brought down the deaths from breast cancer by around 60 per cent in most developed countries. Nearly ten years later, the figures for deaths from breast cancer are still falling, although the numbers detected on screening are, if anything, higher than before. This is a huge forward step in cancer detection and management, and if screening for prostate cancer could do the same for men it would be at least as beneficial, if not more so. So Chapter 8 is about prostate screening, who should have it, and how it is done.

Before going on to screening in detail, however, it is best to clarify the symptoms that men may develop if they have prostate disease, and how they may mean either BPH or prostate cancer.

# 5

# Explaining the symptoms

## Symptoms of prostate disease – do they indicate cancer or BPH?

First, and most important, if you are over 45 years old and are concerned that you may have prostate cancer, you should be given the opportunity to be screened for it. You may have no symptoms at all, but just wish to make sure that you are not at risk. A father, uncle or brother may have had the disease, or you may just have a friend or colleague with it, and wish to reassure yourself. If you see your doctor, you will have two very quick tests – a rectal examination and a test for prostate-specific antigen (PSA), using blood from a forearm vein. If the two together are negative, you can be reassured, and worry no more. A five-yearly re-examination is probably adequate from then on.

It is different if there are symptoms that indicate that prostate cancer is possible. To understand how they may arise, think back to Chapter 1, which describes where the prostate gland is, and its relationship to the bladder and its outlet tube, the urethra. A tumour (growing mass) inside the prostate can compress the urethra and interfere with the delicate nerve and muscle mechanisms at the base of the bladder – and in doing so may hinder the fast and strong flow of urine from the bladder to the penis. As the tumour grows larger, it can extend beyond the normal boundaries of the prostate gland, invading into other structures within the pelvis. For example, it can grow into the bladder itself, to cause blood in the urine, or it can compress the ureter, the tube from the kidney to the bladder, causing pain running from the loin (in the small of the back) to the groin.

Then small parts of the tumour can break away from it, to be deposited in distant parts of the body, such as the bones of the spine and pelvis. This can lead to back pain, anaemia, tiredness and listlessness, along with weight loss, as the cancer deposits (they are called metastases) use up vital energy stores.

Experts in prostate cancer therefore divide the symptoms of prostate disease into three groups:

• symptoms of bladder outflow obstruction;
• symptoms caused by local extension of the tumour into the surrounding pelvic tissues; and
• symptoms caused by distant spread of the cancer.

## Bladder outflow symptoms

There are seven main symptoms of bladder outflow problems:

• poor stream of urine;
• hesitancy (difficulty in starting to pass urine);
• sensation of incomplete emptying after passing urine;
• intermittency (stopping and starting during urination);
• frequency (having to pass urine more often than before – but not necessarily more urine at a time);
• urgency (having to pass urine urgently because of a sudden need that is hard to control); and
• urge incontinence (wetting yourself because you have not been able to reach the toilet in time).

It must be said here that none of these symptoms is exclusive to prostate cancer. They are shared with BPH. Some are also caused by a condition called irritable bladder, in which the nervous system that the bladder uses to detect that it is becoming full is too sensitive, and makes you feel that it is full when it is still half empty. But if you have these symptoms, you must have your prostate checked, because you cannot ignore them.

## The International Prostate Scoring System

These symptoms of bladder outflow problems are so well recognized that the American Urological Association has established an International Prostate Scoring Symptom Score (IPSS), which has been endorsed by the World Health Organization for use in diagnosis and in clinical trials. The IPSS is an excellent way to measure the severity of any urinary obstruction and bladder floor irritation in prostate cancer, and to assess the response to treatments. The IPSS is fully explained here, so you can use it yourself and judge your own progress for yourself.

### The first six questions – bladder outflow problems

Bear in mind that you should give each of the first six questions a score from 0 to 5:

- 0 = not at all
- 1 = less than one time in five
- 2 = less than half the time
- 3 = about half the time
- 4 = more than half the time
- 5 = almost always.

These first six questions all relate to how you have been in the past month.

1  *Incomplete emptying:* How often have you had a sensation of not emptying your bladder completely after you finish urination?
2  *Frequency:* How often have you had to urinate again less than two hours after you finished urinating?
3  *Intermittency:* How often have you found you stopped and started again several times when you urinated?
4  *Urgency:* How often have you found it difficult to postpone urination?
5  *Weak stream:* How often have you had a weak urinary flow or stream?

6 *Straining:* How often have you had to push or strain to start urinating?

Question 7 is scored slightly differently. It is:

Over the past month, how many times did you most typically get up to urinate from the time you went to bed at night to the time you got up in the morning? This time the reply must be chosen from the following:

- 0 = none
- 1 = once
- 2 = twice
- 3 = three times
- 4 = four times
- 5 = five times or more.

## Quality of life

This final question is: If you were to spend the rest of your life with your urinary condition the way it is now, how would you feel about that? Score it as follows:

- 0 = delighted
- 1 = pleased
- 2 = mostly satisfied
- 3 = mixed – about equally satisfied and dissatisfied
- 4 = mostly dissatisfied
- 5 = unhappy
- 6 = terrible.

You will see that you can score from 0 (no problems at all) to 35 (worst of all) on the first seven questions, and from 0 to 6 on the last one. On the symptom score, 0 to 7 is considered mild, 8 to 19 moderate, and 20 to 35 severe. Repeat scoring over months after the start of treatment can give researchers (and, for that matter, yourself) a good idea of how well you are responding to treatment, and how effective the treatment is. It has the extra advantage that the numbers can be used by statisticians to evaluate results in large scale trials of new treatments.

The quality-of-life score, which remains separate from the symptom score, is mostly used as a basis for discussion between patient and doctor about management of the illness and how to improve it. A good quality-of-life score, for example, influences the decision on whether or not your doctor contemplates surgery or other radical treatments, or whether to leave well alone until the quality of life deteriorates.

## Prostate cancer versus BPH

Although the IPSS is useful, it does not help to differentiate prostate cancer from BPH. Because so many men have BPH, most men with prostate cancer also have some degree of BPH, and the outflow symptoms are more likely to be caused by the BPH than the cancer itself. As mentioned in Chapter 1, BPH usually arises in the transition zone close to the urethra, and is therefore more likely to put pressure on the urinary outflow than prostate cancer, which arises much more commonly in the peripheral zone, further from the urethra. This is why some men have 'distant' symptoms of prostate cancer without ever having had any trouble with urine flow.

So, unless the tumour has started in the transition zone, or has become very large, early symptoms of bladder outflow problems are more likely to be due to BPH than to cancer. One way to help to differentiate between the two diseases is to divide the bladder outflow symptoms into two types – obstructive and irritative.

Obstructive symptoms, which are caused by the enlarging mass pressing on the urethra, include reduced flow, hesitancy and incomplete emptying. They are more likely to be due to cancer than to BPH (although they can be caused by either).

The ultimate obstruction is urinary retention, in which urine flow stops, the bladder over-fills, and the patient has a distended abdomen and severe pain. The harder he tries to expel urine, the worse it gets. The only answer is to pass a catheter (a sterile hollow flexible tube) up through the penis past the obstruction, or through the front of the lower abdomen (suprapubic catheterization), to empty the bladder.

Irritative symptoms include frequency and urgency. They are the result of the expanding mass in the prostate pressing up against the base of the bladder, interfering with the delicate 'detrusor' muscle system that co-ordinates and controls the emptying of the bladder as it begins to stretch with a full load of urine. The detrusor system is the one that gives you the message that your bladder needs to empty. You can ignore it for a while, but it returns with its message as the need becomes more urgent. A mass just below the detrusor stretches it, fooling it into believing that the bladder is fuller than it is. Hence the frequency and urgency. Irritative symptoms are commoner with BPH than with prostate cancer, but, like obstructive symptoms, both conditions can cause them.

Bladder outflow symptoms can lead to complications beyond the prostate. For example, a 'pool' of urine left in the bladder after incomplete emptying can easily become infected: it is a perfect place for germs such as bacteria to multiply. This can lead to pain in the bladder (which you feel in the lower half of the abdomen, between the navel and the pelvis), much more frequency and urgency, and pain on passing urine (this is called dysuria). Such infections may lead to obvious blood in the urine. If you pass blood in the urine it is just as likely to be due to infection as to a bleeding tumour, so do not assume the worst. But do report it to your doctor.

This static pool of urine in the bladder is also a perfect medium in which stones can form. These stones, or calculi, are made of calcium particles or of crystals of a waste substance called urate. They can irritate the bladder, again producing pain just above the pelvis and blood in the urine, especially as the act of urination is finishing. Germs find it easy to grow on their surface, so they can also cause urinary infections. Sometimes the first sign of prostate cancer or BPH is the discovery of a stone in the bladder during a straightforward X-ray for pain in the lower abdomen. Any man who is found on X-ray to have such a stone must have his prostate fully investigated. How this is done is explained later.

## Symptoms of local spread

All the symptoms described above relate to men whose tumours have not progressed beyond the boundaries of the prostate gland itself. However, they do overlap a little with the symptoms of the next stage of the disease – spread within the pelvis beyond the prostate. Prostate cancer specialists list nine symptoms typical of prostate cancer that has spread beyond the gland itself, but is still confined within the pelvis. These symptoms are:

- blood in the urine (haematuria);
- pain passing urine (dysuria);
- general lower abdominal pain not linked to passing urine;
- impotence;
- incontinence;
- pain in the loin (the angle between the lowest rib and the spine in the back);
- signs of back pressure of urine on the kidneys;
- severe constipation and bleeding from the rectum; and
- blood in the sperm (haemospermia).

## Why do these symptoms occur?

The blood in the urine in this case comes not from a bladder infection, but from direct invasion of the tumour into the urethra.

The incontinence arises from the tumour invading the 'sphincter' (the muscle at the base of the bladder that closes off to stop the flow of urine into the urethra).

The pain may come from acid urine running over a raw cancer surface in the urethra.

Impotence happens if the tumour invades the complex structures of nerve, blood vessels and muscles that lead to erection.

Extension of the prostate tumour upwards can block urine flow from the kidneys into the bladder, leading to back pressure on the kidneys, and hence the loin pain. As this blockage becomes more severe, the back pressure can damage the kidneys, leading to their eventual failure.

Backwards extension of a prostate tumour may lead to pressure on the bowel that lies just behind it. Some prostate cancers are found in the clinic for rectal disorders, because their only symptoms are of bleeding (it is common for haemorrhoids to be blamed) or a change in the normal bowel habit towards severe constipation.

This sounds a horrific list of symptoms, but it is very rare indeed for any one man to have them all. They are presented here so that you can understand why you have your particular set of symptoms, and to reassure you that they can all be tackled with the correct treatment. Once you know why a symptom has arisen, you are well on the way to devising a solution to it. And that is what all prostate tumour management aims for.

Of course, all of these individual symptoms may arise because of other illnesses. Impotence, for example, is a common accompaniment of diabetes in some older men. It may result from stress, or it may be a side effect of drugs prescribed, for example, for high blood pressure. The important message here is, if you have one or more of these symptoms, to let your doctors know about them, and to be willing to undergo extensive questioning and tests to find out their cause.

## Symptoms of more distant spread

Unfortunately, at the time of their diagnosis, more than half of all men with prostate cancer already show spread of their disease beyond the prostate into the pelvis, and a quarter show spread to distant sites, such as bones. This limits the options for treatment and cure: if they could have been detected earlier they might have been suitable for a more comprehensive attack on their tumours. The only way to do this in the future will be by accurate screening for early prostate cancers, the pros and cons of which are discussed at length in Chapter 8.

The distant tumours are known as metastases, and the symptoms of this more distant spread arise both from local effects at the site at which the cancer cells have lodged and from the general malaise that they cause. How the symptoms affect men with metastases is listed here. The first six are the result of metastases at a particular site:

- bone pain;
- spontaneous fractures (breaks) of bones;
- weakness, numbness or paralysis of a leg;
- enlarged glands in the groin or elsewhere;
- swelling of the legs; and
- pain in the loin.

The last three symptoms arise from the effects of the metastases on general health:

- lethargy and listlessness;
- weight loss; and
- bleeding from skin and bowel.

## Bone problems

Bones, in particular, are the sites of metastases, so they often cause pain in a rib, the pelvis or a long bone such as in the arm or leg. However, the most common pain of distant spread from prostate cancer is in the spine in the back. The start of pain low in the back that does not ease with rest is a fundamental sign of prostate cancer that has spread beyond the pelvis.

Sometimes the invasion of prostate cancer cells into the bones can make them vulnerable to fractures, especially if you bear weight upon them. A broken hip in an elderly man who may have had some urinary outflow problems must be considered a case of prostate cancer unless proved otherwise.

Pain in the back due to prostate cancer deposits in spinal bones can lead, if untreated, to collapse of the relevant vertebra, and this in turn can put pressure on the nerves that run into the spinal cord above and below the collapse, and on the spinal cord itself. This 'spinal cord compression', in which there is pain or numbness and weakness, leading even to paralysis, in the legs, can even be the very first sign of prostate cancer in some men. Any sign of persistent unusual back pain in an older man, especially if there is weakness or numbness, must be treated as an emergency. Removing the activity of the cancer cells (by 'androgen deprivation', by radiotherapy or surgery, as described in Chapter 12) can lead to dramatic improvement in the pain and other symptoms, and can prevent paralysis.

Extension of the tumour into the bone marrow, where the blood is produced, interferes with the production of new red blood cells, leading to anaemia.

## Cancer spread and lymph glands

Cancer cells spread along 'lymph channels' via the groin and alongside the inferior vena cava (the main vein from the abdomen and the lower body to the heart). Lymph glands (much like the tonsils in the throat) that are stationed along the lymph channels react to the cancer cells with an 'immune response', so that they swell and become much firmer. They become most noticeable, of course, when they are near the skin, and that means, for spread from the prostate, glands in the groin are usually the first to show the problem. They become obviously enlarged and very firm, but are not necessarily painful.

Normally these lymph glands in the groin are on the lymph drainage path from the legs back into the body. Lymph is the fluid in which all our tissues are bathed. It constantly flows in lymph channels from the tissues to the centre of the body, where they eventually empty into the main veins to the heart. At regular intervals along the lymph channels are lymph nodes, or lymph glands, that contain masses of white cells called lymphocytes. These lymphocytes act as protectors and filters against inflammation and infection, and also against cancer cells. Cancer cells that enter the lymph system meet up with the lymphocytes in the lymph nodes, where they cause inflammatory reactions that lead to the swellings that are noticed, initially, in the groin.

In this fight to the death between the cancer cells and the lymphocytes, the flow of lymph from the legs may be blocked within the enlarged glands, and lymph builds up in the leg beneath. This leads to a swollen leg, the swelling extending from groin to foot, the medical name for which is lymphoedema.

Men with this stage of the disease usually also show, on specialized X-ray or ultrasound examinations, similarly enlarged glands along the line of the inferior vena cava to the right of the spine inside the abdomen. Some of them may be so large that they press upon the ureter from the kidney on that side – and that can cause back pressure on the kidney, leading to a persistent dull ache in the loin. Later in the spread, if it is not checked, glands may appear as far from the prostate gland as the armpit or neck.

## The relevance of spread of your cancer

Why is it so important to know if your cancer has spread, and to which sites? In the past, a diagnosis of metastatic prostate cancer was disastrous. Little could be done to stop a steady progression to terminal illness and death from the disease. Now, however, we have many ways in which we can arrest the disease, and the treatment and long-term management depends on an accurate diagnosis not just that the cancer exists, but also of where it is, its extent and its susceptibility to each of the treatments that we can use against it.

So if you have been told your cancer has spread, it is no longer a death sentence. It is a challenge for both you and your doctors, but it is one that is very worthwhile taking up. Writing in 2010, and as a practising family doctor in a rural area of south-west Scotland, I know of at least eight men who were given the diagnosis of metastatic prostate cancer before 2000 and who are still well. One is now 74 and can still outdrive me at golf. Thankfully, his putting lets him down now, so I have a chance against him – but that is to do with his eyesight, and not his cancer. There is every reason for you, if you have been given the same diagnosis, to try to emulate these men. Your doctors will surely help you in doing just that.

Their first task in doing so is to find out how extensive your prostate cancer is: in effect, they will 'stage' your tumour. How that is done is the subject of the next chapter.

# 6

# Staging and assessing your tumour

We stage prostate cancers in different ways. The first task of doctors is simply to perform the routine examination that they learned as students and have perfected with experience. This examination involves looking for lumps in the groin, tapping (percussing one finger against another lying flat on the abdominal surface) for an over-full bladder, looking at the legs for swelling and then placing a finger in the rectum.

## The rectal examination and staging of prostate cancer

The rectal examination is still the best way for the experienced doctor to assess the prostate. In the UK it is done with the man lying on his left side, the knees drawn up to the chest. In the USA it is usually performed with the man standing, and leaning forward against a wall. Some doctors now employ a knee–elbow position, on the grounds that it gives a better 'feel' of the whole prostate gland. As most tumours arise in the peripheral zone – that is, the part of the gland that is nearest the finger – rectal examination is remarkably accurate in detecting cancers.

The earliest stage that can be detected is a firm nodule, like a hard pea, that is well within the gland, not altering its shape. This is defined as stage T2a or B1, depending on the system used by the clinic. (Stage T1 is a cancer usually found almost by accident, during tests for BPH, with no indication of tumour on rectal examination. It is described below, in the section on trans-urethral resection of the prostate, or TURP.)

Stage T2b or B2 cancers feel harder still and are larger and more diffuse, with a less well-defined edge, but they remain localized to one side of the gland. Stage T3 (or C) cancers are larger still, and distort the normal prostate outline, but the gland remains mobile and unfixed to the surrounding tissues. Stage T4 (D) cancers lead to a hard, misshapen, enlarged prostate that is much less mobile because it is fixed to the surrounding pelvic structures. They are the cancers most likely to be linked to distant metastases.

## Other conditions detected by rectal examination

Experienced family doctors and all specialists in prostate gland disease can usually tell the difference between cancers and BPH by the 'feel' of the prostate surface and its texture. BPH feels softer and has more 'give' in it than cancer, and the swelling of the gland is much more symmetrical than cancerous masses.

However, there are other prostate conditions that are more easily confused with cancer. One is chronic prostatitis.

Chronic prostatitis is the result of recurrent infections (acute prostatitis) in the prostate gland. These bouts of acute prostatitis are fairly easy to diagnose. They involve all the usual signs of infection, such as fevers, sweating and pain in the lower abdomen. The acute illness also causes severe pain on passing urine, sometimes with blood in the urine, and can be mistaken for a urinary infection. However, the give-away sign is a very tender, but soft, prostate on rectal examination. Doctors have to be very careful doing rectal examinations in men with acute prostatitis, as it can produce extremely severe pain.

The treatment for acute prostatitis is the appropriate antibiotic, but in some cases the infection lingers on. That can eventually lead to hard deposits of calcium (sometimes giving a gritty feeling, or even presenting like a prostate 'stone') that may feel like a cancer. Chronic prostatitis often accompanies BPH, so that the gland is enlarged, too, making confusion with cancer even more likely.

Most of the time the rectal examination alone is enough to confirm or rule out prostate cancer, but there are cases when it is impossible to differentiate between chronic prostatitis and prostate cancer. This is one reason for all suspected cases to be subjected to biopsy – a piece of the prostate is removed and examined under the microscope.

## Biopsy

Experts in prostate diagnosis can use their finger in the rectal examination to guide a fine needle into the gland. Biopsy needles are made so that they can take a piece of material (the biopsy) from the precise site of the abnormality. However, doing it using the finger only is not always easy, so that most biopsies are now taken under the guidance of an ultrasound scan. An ultrasound probe is inserted into the rectum, and an automatic device removes the biopsy during the scan. This is called trans-rectum ultrasound, or TRUS for short. In most prostate units today every suspicious area of prostate is subjected to TRUS biopsy. In fact, TRUS biopsies are also performed in men who have been found at screening (perhaps because of a high prostate-specific antigen – see Chapter 7) to be at high risk of prostate cancer, even if there are no suspicious areas on rectal examination. TRUS may find early lesions that cannot be felt by even the most experienced finger.

## Trans-urethral resection of the prostate (TURP)

Sometimes the diagnosis of prostate cancer is made incidentally after surgery for BPH. Some men with bladder outflow symptoms (see Chapter 5) have, on rectal examination, obvious BPH, and there is no sign of prostate cancer on rectal examination. They are then offered trans-urethral resection of the prostate, or TURP for short.

The best way to describe TURP in layman's language is that the enlarged piece of prostate around the urethra (in the transition zone – see Chapter 1) is 'bored out' by passing a flexible instrument up the urethra into the region of the prostate. It then rotates, and cutting blades are used to remove, in slices, or chippings, the overgrown prostate tissue that is causing the obstruction. The pieces of tissue that are removed during TURP are collected and viewed under a microscope for any signs of malignancy.

Between 10 and 20 per cent of men undergoing TURP for apparently benign prostate disease have traces of cancer in their TURP chippings. These are the stage T1 (or A) cancers described above. They are divided into T1a (A1) and T1b (A2). In T1a disease the tumour cells have a less malignant appearance and occupy less than 5 per cent of the chippings. In T1b disease more than 5 per cent of the chippings show cancerous changes, and they look more malignant.

## Why stage?

Why should we bother to stage prostate cancers, and what can we do with the information? Staging is crucial to the decision on how, or even whether, to proceed with treatment. There is no need for me to remind you that if you are told you have prostate cancer you will be devastated. Yet this is not always the case. I've known men be grateful for at last knowing what was wrong, after months of feeling generally unwell. Even though they had to face up to the fact they had cancer, it was better than not knowing. Now that they had a tangible enemy to fight, they felt better. They felt better still when they started their treatment, and the activity of their cancers began to wane, almost instantaneously.

Not every man needs treatment. In men over 75, the staging process may indicate that the cancer is unlikely to spread quickly or to cause serious problems for many years. They may not need any active treatment, but rather a follow-up examination every year or so, to make sure things have not changed for the worse and that treatment need not yet be started. For men younger than 75, who could fairly be expected to live at least another five years, then accurate staging and appropriate treatment may help to prevent their disease from developing further and from metastasizing. Staging can identify the men who will benefit most from the different forms of treatment that can now be offered to them. They are described in the last part of this book.

However, before we turn to treatments, we need first to understand the subject of 'tumour markers' and how their level in the blood affects how we treat and follow up men with prostate cancer. The one we use today is prostate-specific antigen, but more are to come.

# 7

# Prostate-specific antigen (PSA)

Doctors would like to have a tumour marker for every cancer. A tumour marker is a simple blood test that shows us how active a cancer is, even when the patient is still feeling well and has no symptoms. Then the disease can be treated before it gives symptoms, and may even be kept under complete control. We do have one for prostate cancer – prostate-specific antigen, or PSA.

Technically speaking, PSA is a glycoprotein, a compound of protein and sugar that is formed only by the cells in the lining of the prostatic ducts, the tiny tubes that carry the prostatic fluid to the urethra. Its normal function in the body is to break down proteins formed in the seminal vesicles, small sacs at the back of the prostate in which sperm from the testicles collects. Although most PSA remains within the prostate, some 'spills over' into the bloodstream. PSA levels in prostatic fluid, for example, are one million times higher than those in the blood, but still this 'spill-over' PSA can be measured, very accurately, in blood taken from a vein.

## PSA in the diagnosis of prostate cancer

There were early problems devising an assay (a method for measuring PSA), but the newest methods are extremely reliable. Higher than normal blood PSA levels occur in prostate cancer, and not in any other form of cancer. In most men with no prostate disease, the PSA is less than four nanograms per millilitre (ng/ml). The figures do rise with age, but even in extreme old age, in men without prostate cancer, PSA levels are hardly ever above ten ng/ml in most laboratory assay systems.

PSA levels also rise, and stay high for two weeks, after needle biopsies of the prostate are taken, after TURP (see Chapter 6), and even after catheters and other instruments are passed into the urethra. They are therefore usually measured either before your surgeon performs any of these procedures, or at least a fortnight afterwards.

Moderate rises in PSA (to around 20 ng/ml) may be recorded in men with BPH or prostatitis, and in the early stages (T1a and T1b) of prostate cancer, but the bigger rises, of 50 to 800 ng/ml, are found in more advanced cancers (stage T4). The main reason for a steep rise in PSA, therefore, is active prostate cancer. This is why PSA measurement was originally approved in the USA and Europe, including the UK, for use in following the progress of men with known prostate cancer. More recently its use has been extended to early cancer detection and screening.

PSA levels relate quite closely to the stage of the cancer. Doctors from Stanford University Hospital in California have shown that each gram of prostate cancer tissue adds 3.5 ng/ml to the blood PSA level. Values above ten ng/ml usually mean that the cancer has spread beyond the limits of the normal gland. However, this does not necessarily mean distant metastases. The Mayo Clinic Prostate Cancer Group reported that only one of 306 men with proven prostate cancer and PSA levels below 20 ng/ml at initial diagnosis had positive bone scans for metastatic cancer.

## PSA in assessing treatment effects and outlook

PSA is therefore valuable in the initial diagnosis, in that it reflects how much active cancer there is, and whether it may have spread. It is also helpful in judging how well treatment has worked. For example, within a few weeks of starting successful treatment, PSA values should fall steeply, towards near zero. Most men with undetectable PSA levels after, for example, a radical prostatectomy (surgery to remove the whole prostate in men with no spread beyond the gland itself) remain disease-free permanently. They can be considered cured of their cancers. In the few whose PSA subsequently rises again, this is the first sign of a recurrence of their disease, and it indicates that further treatment may be needed to prevent spread.

In one report of 230 men followed for four years after radical prostatectomy, only 41 eventually showed a rise in PSA. Eighty-two per cent of the men with rising PSA survived another five years and 72 per cent survived for more than ten years after the PSA rise. These are good figures for men most of whom were already elderly when they underwent their operations. They show that a rising PSA is not necessarily a death sentence: it may show that some cancer remains, but that it is not aggressive enough even to cause symptoms, far less threaten life. This is something to remember if you are told that your PSA has risen a little.

The aim of radical prostatectomy is to remove all the cancer in the prostate at one operation. It is done only in men whose cancer is thought to be confined to the gland itself, not having spread beyond the edges of the gland either into the pelvis or into distant sites. So it is always done in hope of a complete cure. The figures above suggest that it often fulfils that hope. When the cancers have spread beyond the prostate, either locally or distantly, then radical prostatectomy is not an option. Surgery can no longer clear the disease, and might spread it further. So the next choice is between radiation therapy (radiotherapy) and hormonal (anti-androgen) therapy. I write about them in Chapter 12. They may not offer cure, but they can arrest the progress of the disease – and the PSA measurement helps to confirm or not whether they have done so.

Radiotherapy is usually offered to men whose disease may have spread locally in the pelvis so far that its complete surgical removal is impossible. PSA levels fall dramatically after successful radiotherapy. In 1989, the Stanford group in the USA followed men after radiotherapy: 82 per cent of them showed a significant drop in PSA over the next year. This is now more than 20 years ago: progress in radiation techniques since then (we can focus the radiation much more closely now, using radium needles) must have improved upon these figures. Other groups have shown that men whose PSA levels drop steeply after radiation do very well for many years afterwards. The converse is that a PSA that does not fall, or starts to rise, after radiation therapy tends to suggest persistent cancer – and such cancer has to be treated further. The usual alternative is anti-hormone, or anti-androgen, treatment.

You will be offered anti-androgen treatment if at the time of diagnosis your cancer has already spread to distant organs (metastasis). It is also used either along with, or after, radiotherapy, particularly if PSA levels have not fallen enough to rule out remaining active disease. A fall in PSA to levels near the norm (preferably under ten ng/ml, and even better to under one ng/ml) is a good sign of response to anti-androgen therapy. In one study of 48 men with metastases from prostate cancer, those whose PSA levels fell below four ng/ml had a much longer period free of recurrence than those whose PSAs remained high. This study also showed that a rise in PSA could be noted an average of seven months before any new symptoms arose, giving doctors and the men themselves time to prepare for further treatments.

## Summary

To summarize, PSA is invaluable in:

- diagnosing prostate cancer;
- helping to 'stage' the disease; and
- monitoring the results of treatment.

You will continue to need repeat tests for the rest of your life. This may sound daunting, and even frightening, in that you may always be fearful of it rising again and worried about what may happen when it does. But for most men it is reassuring, because each time they hear that it has stayed at its normal level, they can be happy that their disease is no longer active. That means a lot.

One use of PSA, however, needs a special chapter of its own. In the USA, it is used to 'screen' apparently healthy men for the earliest stages of prostate cancer. Should this practice be adopted elsewhere? On the surface, it would seem to be of great benefit, but the concept of screening for cancer is still a matter for debate. If you are reading this book because someone close to you has prostate cancer, and you are worried that you may yourself develop it, then you may have thought about going for a prostate cancer screen. Please read the next chapter before you do so. It puts forward the current arguments for and against screening. There are pros and cons to discovering that you have an early prostate cancer.

# 8

# Screening for prostate cancer

I have to say here that I am for cancer screening. I am sure as a doctor that if I have patients, male or female, who are in the early stages of a cancer that has not yet grown large enough to cause the symptoms that would bring it to their notice, I would like to know about it. It is a general rule that the earlier we can detect a cancer, the greater the chance we have of curing it completely.

This is certainly true of breast cancer in women. By 2001, we had had breast cancer screening in western Europe for around 30 years. For most of that time, arguments raged about whether it was useful. Did inviting all women aged 45 and older to have mammograms really reduce deaths from breast cancer? The answer was a long time in coming, but it was worth it when it did. As is often the case in medicine, the Scandinavians came up with the proof. Since they started breast cancer screening, breast cancer deaths among the women who came for screening have dropped to less than half of those in women who did not. The drop in deaths was a staggering 63 per cent. The difference was not because women who came for screening had fewer cancers: it was because the cancers were caught so early that they were much more likely to be cured. Those 2001 figures were so convincing that the arguments about screening for breast cancer stopped. We were all convinced of its usefulness. Nearly ten years later, the continuing benefits are even clearer. The fall in breast cancer deaths have continued year by year as fewer and fewer women have died from breast cancer, even though more cases have been brought to light by the screening.

53

In 2001 I wrote in the first edition of this book that the same could be done for prostate cancer, but that the benefits, if they exist, will not be shown for many years – perhaps 15 years or more. For me that was not a reason to hold back. I thought that it should be started then. However, in trying to be unbiased about the question of screening for prostate cancer, I gave the two sides of the argument then. In the next few pages I repeat what I wrote then: I have added, however, the state of play, so to speak, on screening as published in the autumn of 2009 in two major medical journals, the *British Medical Journal* and the *Lancet*. If you are reading this book because you fear you may develop prostate cancer, please read the whole chapter.

## Screening – the view from 2001

First we must define screening. It is a process whereby doctors or other members of the primary health-care team (often nurses) invite apparently well people to have a health check. The people chosen for the invitation are taken from the medical list, are usually from a particular age group, and have not had a recent examination for the problem to be screened. The aim is to find, if possible, signs of serious disease before it becomes obvious because symptoms have appeared. Simple examples are checks for high blood pressure or for diabetes, which only involve a cuff around the arm or a urine test. These screening methods are relatively cheap and can lead to worthwhile health benefits because both conditions can be treated very satisfactorily.

Breast cancer screening is more complex, because it involves mammography. This entails an X-ray of each breast. It can often be very painful, because the breast must be compressed for the X-ray between two plates, but most women tolerate it in order to be assured that their breasts are healthy. Mammography is now proved to be more accurate than self-examination for breast lumps: it detects lumps that are too small to be detected by the woman's own hands. The big advantage in finding such small breast cancers is that we now know that there is a big advantage in doing so: treated so early, they are much less likely to lead to the woman's early death.

Screening for prostate cancer is more complex. First of all it involves a digital rectal examination. This is not pleasant. Coupled with the fact that men are more reluctant than women to go to their doctors when they are well, the thought of a rectal examination is a powerful disincentive to them to accept their doctors' invitations for a health check. PSA is also part of the screen, but some men just do not wish to know whether or not they may have cancer – the thought of such an accurate blood test frightens them, and they avoid it.

However, the third reason against screening comes from some of my colleagues. They feel that making the diagnosis of prostate cancer too early simply complicates men's lives without offering them any advantages. Most prostate cancers, they argue, will grow so slowly that they will never need treatment. So why give such a serious diagnosis to someone who really does not need to know? They believe that it is cruel and unnecessary, and they do have a point.

My problem with that argument is that it does not take into account the men whose prostate cancers will need treatment if we are to save their lives. Is it ethical to ignore them because we are trying not to upset the others whose cancers are not going to kill them?

The fact remains that if we wait to detect prostate cancers in men until they develop symptoms such as bladder outflow problems, or back pain due to spread of the cancer, we are consigning many of them to years of ill-health. Without screening, fewer than one in three men are candidates for cure at the moment of their diagnosis, and only one in ten has such minimal and slowly growing cancer that it does not need treatment. This leaves a majority for whom treatment aims to arrest, rather than to cure, the cancer process.

With properly organized screening, we should be able to identify many more men at much earlier stages of their cancers, when we can do something radical about them. We should at the same time try to decrease the numbers of cases and to improve the effectiveness of prostate cancer treatment.

Reducing the numbers of cases may not be so far fetched. Although we do not know why men develop prostate cancer, we do know that the drug finasteride (it is one of a group of drugs called 5-alpha-reductase inhibitors) will shrink the swollen tissues of prostate glands affected by BPH. It is now the standard treatment of BPH. Some researchers have proposed that it may also prevent the initial stages of prostate cancer, and a large-scale trial of finasteride in the possible prevention of prostate cancer was set up to test this hypothesis in the USA in 2000. Unfortunately, by 2010 there was no definite evidence that it might do so. It is still hoped that wide use of this drug in men with BPH will eventually lower their prostate cancer rates.

As for improving the treatment of prostate cancer once it is diagnosed, this may be more difficult. Put simply, we have radical prostatectomy, radiotherapy and cryotherapy (freezing) for cancers confined to the prostate, radiotherapy for cancers that have spread a little more widely, and anti-hormone treatment for cancers that have spread to distant sites. All are effective treatments, and even if they do not cure the cancers outright they often keep them at bay for years. Naturally, researchers are constantly seeking still more effective treatments.

So, if we already have reasonably successful treatments for prostate cancer, and it is a relatively common disease, why do we not screen for it much more widely? The answer lies in some unique characteristics of prostate cancer. It is alone among cancers of any other organ in that it is far more common than could ever be imagined from the numbers of men in whom it causes symptoms. When prostate glands are examined at post-mortem examination of men who have died from other causes, very many more of them than could be expected contain areas of cancer. In 1985, for example, 86,000 American men were diagnosed as having prostate cancer. This was only around one per cent of the eight million men in whom prostate cancers, quite unexpectedly, were found at post-mortem examination in the same year.

It was worked out that the risk of developing this form of 'autopsy cancer', as it was called in the USA, during an average man's lifetime, was as high as 42 per cent. This was in contrast to a lifetime risk of developing clinical prostate cancer (cancer that causes symptoms and illness) of nine per cent, and a lifetime risk of dying from such a prostate cancer of only 2.9 per cent. Put another way, only three men in a thousand with areas of cancer in their prostates actually die from the disease.

If screening for prostate cancer detects all of these cases, then what should be done with this knowledge? Treating them all with anticancer therapy would be like taking a sledge-hammer to crack a nut, a form of 'overkill' in which far too many men would be treated unnecessarily to save the lives of a small minority. And treatment for prostate cancer does have unwanted effects.

So if screening is to be effective it should detect only those cancers that will progress to produce illness and perhaps death, and leave undetected those that will remain low-key and unthreatening. This is not easy. We have to produce a system that detects the cancers before they cause the first symptoms, but they must only be those that we consider will cause those symptoms in the near future. By the time they have caused symptoms, the disease is often already past the stage of possible cure, and this is no longer 'screening'.

Can this be done satisfactorily with the methods we have at our disposal today? To some extent, yes. We have three screening methods:

- digital rectal examination (use of the doctor's finger), or DRE;
- rectal ultrasound; and
- prostate-specific antigen, or PSA.

Probably the best review of the effectiveness of these methods in detecting early cancers that need treatment is by Dr Michael K. Brawer of Seattle, one of the authors of the best doctor's book on prostate cancer, *Prostate Cancer*, published by Elsevier.

The Seattle team reported that neither DRE nor rectal ultrasound were particularly accurate, taken on their own, in detecting early cancers. Ultrasound was the more effective of the two, but it is too costly and not accurate enough to detect early cancers in a mass screening of an apparently healthy population of men. Nevertheless, the team agreed that trans-rectal ultrasound that uses a spring-loaded needle to take biopsies from a suspicious area within the prostate is the most accurate way to make the diagnosis.

PSA on its own, too, is less accurate in detecting early prostate cancer than was hoped. One problem, for example, is where to put the dividing line between a normal PSA and one that indicates abnormal prostate activity that might be cancer. In screening studies defining PSA levels above four ng/ml as abnormal and below four ng/ml as a sign that the prostate was normal, about 2 per cent were in the abnormal range. Around one-third of this 2 per cent turned out, on further examination using an ultrasound-guided biopsy needle, to have prostate cancer. So using PSA alone will detect just under one cancer case in a hundred healthy men screened. Whether all the cases detected in this way should be treated is still a matter for debate.

Dr Brawer's Seattle team went further. They took PSA tests from an initial number of 1249 apparently healthy men over the age of 50 for three years. Their aim was to see what happened to the men in whom the PSA was rising, year by year. Each year they asked the men whose PSA levels had increased by 20 per cent over the previous year's result to have a biopsy of their prostates. They reasoned that an annual increase of 20 per cent in PSA was a reliable sign that there may be an actively growing cancer. Other studies had shown that PSA in men with prostate cancer doubles every four to five years.

Using this method of a steadily increasing PSA each year, the Seattle group detected prostate cancer in around 2 per cent of their original group each year. In actual numbers, 14 men in the first year, 12 in the second year and 13 in the third year had prostate cancers that needed curative treatment. This must be considered a good result for these men, whose future quality of life must have been greatly improved by their good fortune in having their cancers detected so early. However, Dr Brawer warns that a significant proportion (perhaps as high as one in six) of men with prostate cancers have PSA levels under four ng/ml at the time of diagnosis.

He mentions another worry. In the past, many men were found to have prostate cancer incidentally when they were having trans-urethral resection of the prostate (TURP) for BPH. Their cancers were only discovered when the 'chippings' from their TURP were examined under the microscope. This opportunity for discovering cancer early is being diminished because many fewer cases of BPH are now being treated by TURP. Instead, the routine is to give them the drug finasteride mentioned above, to 'shrink' the enlarged gland, before considering TURP. Is this medical innovation, much welcomed by doctors and patients alike because it avoids or at least postpones the need for surgery, going to leave some early cancers undetected until they have spread?

This does seem possible, because the Seattle group found that 13 per cent of 91 men waiting for TURP because of symptoms of bladder outlet obstruction, who were thought to have only BPH, were found also to have prostate cancer with real potential for causing serious illness. Admittedly they all had an asymmetrical enlarged prostate or a PSA above four ng/ml. These figures are a lesson for doctors to be aware of the possibility of cancer in every man thought to have BPH. All men with BPH should be screened, using rectal ultrasound (with biopsy where appropriate) and PSA, for prostate cancer.

## Summary

To summarize the usefulness of screening for prostate cancer:

- Doctors are improving their DRE, rectal ultrasound and biopsy techniques for detecting early prostate cancer.
- PSA measurements are accurate, and a 'cut-off' point of four ng/ml is a reasonable one above which one should investigate for cancer.
- Repeated PSA tests that show a rise, year on year, are suggestive of active cancer.
- DRE and PSA together do detect early cancers that will probably cause severe disease.

The results of doctors like the Seattle team in screening have led to prostate screening becoming almost as common as breast screening in the USA. It may only be coincidence, but since screening started there, numbers of prostate cancer deaths among Americans have fallen for the first time (and have continued to fall in the ten years after the Seattle team's results). In the Mayo Clinic in Rochester, Minnesota and in Stanford, California there has been a big shift from cases of stage T3 disease to stage T1 disease at diagnosis. This is a shift from incurable to curable cancers and is a welcome sign that the screening programme has brought results.

## Problems with screening

However, it is one thing to diagnose prostate cancer earlier, but quite another to show that doing so leads to more effective treatment, saving lives and improving the quality of life. There are many reports of untreated men with known prostate cancer whose cancers never progressed to their final stages: some older men with prostate cancer are better left untreated. That has to be balanced against the 3 per cent of men who do eventually die from their prostate cancer and who must at one stage have had early curable disease. Had these men been treated in time their deaths might have been avoided.

Large-scale trials are already running with the aim of solving this problem. In Scandinavia, the Swedish Oncology Group (oncology being the study of cancer) is randomly allocating newly diagnosed cases of early prostate cancer to radical prostatectomy (extensive surgical removal of the prostate) or to 'watchful waiting' (that is, not treating them at all). And in Denmark there is a similar trial in which men are being allocated to radiation therapy (using a technique called external-beam radiation) and what is called 'expectant management' (that is, doing nothing until or unless an emergency arises). In the USA the PIVOT trial (it stands for Prostate cancer Intervention Versus Observation Trial) has compared surgery versus no treatment in 1050 American men with clinically localized cancer of the prostate. The recent results (I am writing in 2010) have not shown a significant difference in survival between the two groups, but there is difficulty with the allocation of men to these groups, because many men, understandably, do not wish to be included in the 'no-treatment' group.

Trials are one thing, ordinary medical practice quite another. Who should do the screening for prostate cancer? Central to screening must be the GPs – the family doctors. Given that most men with prostate cancer are getting on in years, and that many may have other illnesses that may shorten their expectation of life, it may not be in their interest to have a prostate cancer diagnosed. As a rule of thumb, most doctors would not screen men for prostate cancer if their life expectancy, because of another illness or their age, is less than ten years.

However, family doctors who wish to screen the older men on their lists will do so very effectively by performing a DRE and taking blood for PSA measurement. If either is suggestive of prostate cancer, then a trans-rectal biopsy will be taken using an ultrasound-guided instrument from suspicious sites within the prostate gland. The screen can be repeated every two or three years. It is done at shorter intervals if the PSA is slightly raised, and is tending to rise further on repeated sampling.

## Screening – the view from 2010

Since I wrote the first edition of this book in 2001, the debate about the need for universal screening has finally been settled, at least in the UK. It has been decided there is no place for universal screening. Instead, in 2009 every general practice in Great Britain and Northern Ireland was sent details of a Prostate Cancer Risk Management Programme, to help men to decide whether or not they should be screened (using PSA and DRE). If you are worried that you might be at high risk of the disease, or that you may already be showing symptoms of it, you can ask your doctor about your risk, knowing that your doctor has the information needed to give an accurate answer. If you still feel that you would like a PSA test, you can ask for one. If you are 50 years old or older, or a younger man with a higher than average risk, you are entitled to it.

I am particularly fortunate as a family doctor to practise in the south-west of Scotland, because in this area the relationships between the GPs and hospital doctors are excellent. They work well for all the specialties, but our urological cancer unit at the Ayr Hospital has a well-deserved extra reputation. So for the 2010 edition of this book I asked Mr Graham Holland, our specialist in prostate cancer, to help me update the facts on testing, and then on treatments. I will return to his advice on treatment later. As for testing, the only real difference in screening from 2001 seems to be that we have lowered the level of PSA at which we begin to suspect that a patient might have prostate cancer.

We now recognize that PSA levels rise with age in the general population, and that a level that used to be perceived as 'normal' may not be so in younger men. A man aged 70 with a 'normal' prostate naturally has a higher PSA than does a man aged 50. We now see 'normality' as a PSA below three ng/ml of blood for men aged 50 to 59, below four ng/ml for men in their 60s, and below five ng/ml for men in their 70s and beyond. This has had the effect of raising the threshold for investigation in older men, but lowering it for younger men. We have also realized that vigorous exercise less than 48 hours before testing puts up the PSA level, so that we now ask men to take things easy for two days before the test. Ejaculation, apparently, has a similar effect, so that if you are about to be tested, please abstain from sex for two days beforehand. Otherwise you may be given a falsely high PSA result.

On 31 October 2009 the *Lancet*, one of the principal international medical journals, published an editorial entitled 'Screening for prostate cancer remains controversial'. Written by David E. Neal and colleagues from the Universities of Cambridge, Bristol and Oxford, it analysed the results of two large trials of screening – the European Randomized Study of Screening for Prostate Cancer (ERSPC) and the Prostate, Lung, Colorectal and Ovarian cancer (PLCO) screening trial. ERSPC concluded that 1410 men would have to be screened and 48 would need treatment to prevent one death.

Dr Neal and his colleagues wrote that PSA testing lacks sensitivity and specificity. The first (lacking sensitivity) means that it can miss some cases of cancer, and the second (lacking specificity) means that it is positive in some illnesses that are not cancer. They add that about one-third of men with a PSA between three and ten ng/ml have prostate cancer, but that there is no lower limit below which we can be certain that there is no cancer. Some men are therefore falsely reassured, from their low PSA, that they have no cancer, but lowering the level of PSA to identify them increases the probability of identifying very low-risk cancers that would not need treatment, and would only worry the patients.

The PLCO trial involved 76,000 men. It was stopped early because there was no difference in the death rates of the two groups (screened and unscreened) after ten years (all the men had been followed for at least seven years). Unfortunately, the news about PSA had led to a substantial number of the men in the unscreened group having PSA tests and rectal examinations during the trial, which means that it will be almost impossible to prove, at least from this trial, that screening is either beneficial or harmful.

We are still waiting for the results of the US PIVOT trial referred to in the 2001 edition of this book, along with the equivalent UK ProtecT study. UK ProtecT has tested more than 110,000 men so far (as of 2010) and is following the progress of more than 1600 men who were found in the trial to have prostate cancer confined to the prostate gland. They have been allocated to monitoring only, radical surgery (total prostatectomy) or radiotherapy. We may need to wait another ten years before we know which treatment is most successful and has the fewest unwanted effects.

These conclusions are naturally disappointing, but as the *Lancet* writers conclude: 'Full counselling for men who request a PSA test remains essential because of the continuing uncertainty. For men with low risk disease we need to refine monitoring protocols to ensure that the opportunity for cure is not lost and patients are not treated unnecessarily.'

How we go about doing this is described in the next chapter.

# 9

# Investigating prostate cancer

Once a prostate cancer is suspected (from rectal examination and prostate-specific antigen, or PSA) it needs to be confirmed. That is usually done by needle biopsy (a small piece of tissue removed through a hollow needle) under the view of an ultrasound probe placed in the rectum – a trans-rectal ultrasound, or TRUS. The tissue is then examined under a microscope and the pattern of the cancer cells is assessed for their potential for slow or fast growth – that is, for its potential to remain as a slow-growing tumour inside the prostate or to become more aggressive and spread outside the gland and into distant tissues such as bone.

## TRUS

TRUS is performed by a urologist, a radiologist or a specialist nurse. About half an hour before it and for several days afterwards you will take an antibiotic to prevent infection passing into the prostate through the injection site. The probe is about the size of a finger: it is lubricated with gel, and passed into the rectum so that the tip lies against the prostate. A needle is passed along the inside of the probe, and through it you will be given a local anaesthetic to prevent pain as the biopsies are taken. This is all done under ultrasound guidance, so that the operator can see exactly where the biopsies are being taken from.

Some men find the biopsies painful, others sense only a minor discomfort: the whole operation takes about 15 minutes. It's usual to wait for half an hour afterwards before you can leave.

## The Gleason score

The microscopic assessment is called the Gleason score. Its intricacies are beyond the scope of this book, but put simply, much depends on whether the tumour cells retain their gland-like appearance and whether they retain well defined borders (in which case the cancer will be less malignant) or whether they become a mass of similar-looking cells with no hint of glands or ducts (which signifies intense malignancy). Gleason scores range from 1 to 10. Their importance is illustrated by the 1994 report of Dr G. W. Chodak and colleagues (*New England Journal of Medicine*, volume 334, page 242), which listed the chance of a tumour with Gleason score of 2–4 causing metastases in the following year as 2.1 per cent per year. This rose to 5.4 per cent with Gleason scores of 5–7, and 13.5 per cent with Gleason scores of 8–10. Most men with prostate cancer turn out to have Gleason scores between 5 and 7.

When the three main ways of assessing prostate cancers (rectal examination, PSA and Gleason score) are put together, they become very accurate not only in staging the cancer at diagnosis but also in helping to predict the long-term outcome, whether it is necessary to treat it at all, and how to treat it once the decision to treat has been made.

## Newer tests

Newer tests to try to refine further these predictions are also outside the remit of this book, because they are not yet routine even in hospitals that specialize in prostate cancer treatment. They are mentioned here, however, to show that progress is being made. One is the assessment of the numbers of new blood vessels within and around the tumour. They correlate to some extent with the ability of the tumour to spread. Another technique looks for tumour cells expressing abnormal genes found only in cancer: this is still a long way from regular use.

The newest TRUS machines will spot problems (the echo of sound returning from tumours differs from the echo received from normal tissues) as small as 0.2 mm in diameter. They can differentiate between normal and abnormal prostate tissues, and show the parts of the gland that are over-endowed with blood vessels. This last indicates either areas of active cancer or areas of inflammation caused by prostatitis.

Some prostate cancer centres are adding magnetic resonance imaging (MRI) to their investigations. MRI uses differences in magnetic fields, rather than X-rays or sound waves, to produce its images, which are remarkably clear. So far, however, comparisons with TRUS have not shown it to be any more accurate in defining the extent of prostate tumours inside or outside the gland, and it is far more expensive.

Computed tomography (CT) scanning is not helpful in assessing disease within the prostate because, unlike TRUS or MRI, CT cannot reveal details of differences in texture or density of tissue inside the gland. It can detect, however, enlarged lymph glands outside the prostate, in the pelvis and higher in the abdomen. Some centres use it when men have PSA levels above 20 ng/ml and a Gleason score more than 7, to see if there is spread into lymph nodes outside the pelvis. If they have, then this makes a difference to the decision on whether or not to operate. If CT scans do identify enlarged lymph glands, they may then be 'dissected out' at surgery. If the affected lymph glands are too extensive for complete dissection, then radiation therapy or anti-hormone therapy will be considered instead.

### Bone scans

To make the investigation complete, the bones may be scanned for metastases. This is done using radionuclides, traces of radioactive elements that are selectively taken up by cancer cells and show as hot spots in the skeleton, usually in the spine and long bones of the arms and legs. Radionuclide scans are not always necessary. More than half of all men with newly diagnosed prostate cancer have PSA levels under ten ng/ml. There is such a small chance that their tumours have spread into bone that radionuclide scanning is no longer thought to be necessary. For example, in one series of 852 men with newly diagnosed prostate cancer and a PSA below ten ng/ml, only seven men had positive scans. Five of the seven already had painful bones that suggested to their doctors before the scan that some spread had occurred (Lee and Oesterling, *Urological Clinics of North America*, 1997, volume 24, page 389). In another series of 290 men with PSA levels below ten ng/ml undergoing radionuclide scans, none had bony spread (Gleave and colleagues, *Urology*, 1996, volume 46, page 708). In yet another study, none of 861 newly diagnosed men with PSA levels below 20 ng/ml had any bony hot spots (Levran and colleagues, *British Journal of Urology*, 1995, volume 75, page 778).

Because of these studies, most prostate cancer specialists order bone scans only when the initial PSA level on diagnosis is above 20 ng/ml, or when there is another reason, such as persistent pain in a particular spot, to suspect bone involvement. If a bone scan does reveal spread of the cancer then it rules out the option of radical prostatectomy, the surgery that removes the whole prostate gland with the aim of curing the disease. Who should be offered radical prostatectomy and what it entails is described in Chapter 11.

# 10

## The decision to treat

After all the tests, which include rectal examination, a measurement of prostate-specific antigen (PSA) and an ultrasound-guided biopsy, what does the prostate team do with the results? That is the subject of this short chapter. To select the correct treatment for each newly diagnosed case of prostate cancer, the specialists use what is called a 'decision tree' based on the PSA and transurethral ultrasound (TRUS) findings.

The decision tree starts with the finding of a raised PSA – levels above four ng/ml need to be further investigated, preferably first with a TRUS biopsy. This gives one of three results:

- The first possible result is a negative result for cancer, and may indicate a low-grade prostate infection (prostatitis). Such cases only need watching over many months to make sure that the PSA is not steadily rising. In prostatitis that responds to antibiotics, the PSA level will return to normal.
- The second possible result is also negative for prostate cancer, but shows a high-grade prostatitis. If this does not resolve on antibiotic treatment, TRUS biopsies will be repeated. The biopsies may eventually be shown to be positive for cancer, or they remain negative. Rising PSA levels tend to indicate cancer.
- The third possible result is a positive finding of cancer. In this case, the PSA level will be assessed along with the Gleason score from the microscope appearance from the biopsy.

It is the third result that concerns us. Men who come under the third category are split into two further groups:

- In one of these groups, those with a PSA below ten ng/ml and a Gleason score of 6 or below, there is very little risk of extension of the cancer beyond the prostate. These patients must discuss with their doctor their treatment options, which, frankly, are to do nothing, or to have a radical prostatectomy or undergo radiation therapy.
- In the other group, those with a PSA above ten ng/ml and a Gleason score of 7 or above, there is a high risk of extension of the cancer beyond the prostate. These patients need to have a radionuclide bone scan. They may also have a CT or MRI scan, although these scans are less necessary or useful in most cases. If they are found to have cancer extended beyond the prostate boundaries, then they, too, must discuss their treatment options with their doctor. Their choice is usually anti-hormone therapy.

All these treatments are described in the next chapters.

# 11

# Treating cancer confined to the prostate gland – surgery

Once the staging process described in the previous chapters has proved that the cancer is still confined to the prostate, there is a need to take action. The aim of treatment in men in this early stage of prostate cancer is cure, if possible, providing that the treatment does offer them a reasonable quality of life for a reasonable number of years. Probably the best definition of the aims of treatment of prostate cancer was given at an International Consensus Workshop on Screening and Global Strategy for Prostate Cancer held in Belgium in 1995. Still relevant today, though it may sound shocking to you, it asked delegates to aim at 'affording the patient the best chance of dying of something else'.

There is considerable truth in this statement. Most men discovered to have prostate cancers confined to the gland will have hardly any, or even no, problems from their cancers for several years. It is not sensible to subject the older men among them, perhaps with other illnesses and a life expectancy less than ten years, to rigorous treatments that will be uncomfortable, to say the least.

So the treatment options for early prostate cancer that has not yet spread must include doing nothing but 'watching and waiting'. If you are offered that option do consider it seriously: it could be the best management for you, and it is not a matter of your specialists opting out of your care. Naturally, you will be asked back regularly for tests for prostate-specific antigen (PSA), rectal examinations and, if necessary, repeat biopsies, to make sure that the tumour is not growing and threatening to spread. Once there are signs that it may start to cause symptoms and worsen your quality of life, treatment can then be started.

Today the treatment options for localized cancers like this are growing year by year. As of 2010, they include:

- trans-urethral resection of the prostate (TURP);
- radical prostatectomy;
- external-beam radiation;
- brachytherapy;
- cryotherapy;
- androgen deprivation; and
- laser therapy.

Some of these treatments aim to eradicate all of the cancer tissue, others, such as androgen deprivation, do not. All of them, however, have the aim of hitting the tumour so hard that it will not threaten the man's life for such a long time that he can expect to have died naturally from other causes before that happens. Drs Kirby, Christmas and Brawer, in their book on prostate cancer published in 2001, made the point that when all these treatments have been compared for men with early prostate cancers (it is difficult to compare them in a completely unbiased way), they have similar success rates. So the choice of the treatment depends at least as much on the quality of life the man enjoys after the treatment has started as on the chances of saving his life.

As of 2010, most specialists still adhere to that viewpoint.

## TURP

To be frank, TURP is an operation designed for BPH, not cancer. It is used only in older men who have bladder outflow symptoms because they have both BPH and a small prostate cancer close to the urethra (that is, in the transition zone, which is the usual site of BPH). It is not an option for prostate cancers in the peripheral zone (the commonest site for cancer) or in men with no bladder outflow problems.

## Radical prostatectomy

Radical prostatectomy was much more widely performed in North America than in the UK or northern Europe until the late 1990s. In my region of Ayrshire, we were fortunate that our prostate surgeons were British pioneers in this operation, having performed radical prostatectomies since 1996, with a rate of around 20 per year by 2003. That is important, because experienced surgeons have lower rates of unwanted after-effects than do those who operate less frequently.

This operation is confined to men in whom there is a good chance of complete cure by removing the whole prostate gland at operation. They therefore must fulfil the following criteria:

- they must have only T1 or T2 disease (disease limited to the prostate gland with no spread outside its capsule);
- they must be closely investigated for possible metastases and spread into the abdomen;
- they must be relatively healthy otherwise, with no signs of serious other diseases; and
- they should have a life expectancy of more than ten years.

These conditions may sound harsh, but the operation is an extensive one, requiring great surgical skill, and the patient may pass through an unpleasant and fairly stormy period immediately after it. It is not one to be contemplated by someone who is older and not in the best of health. On the other hand, if it is a success, it has the huge advantage over other treatments that it gives you the security of knowing that the whole tumour has been removed and will not come back. It is then a true cure and takes much of the anxiety out of the years that follow. It is also a cure for BPH for the many men who have both prostate diseases.

Before the operation you will have a chest X-ray, an electrocardiogram and blood tests to ensure that the kidneys are normal and there is no anaemia. You may be asked to donate two or three units of your own blood beforehand, so that it can be transfused back into you during and after the operation. This is autologous transfusion, and it is being used more often in these days of fears (mostly unfounded in countries like the UK) about contaminated donor blood. Just before the operation you will start taking an antibiotic to prevent infection during surgery from bowel bacteria.

The prostate is removed either through the abdomen or via the perineum, the space between the back of the scrotum and the front of the anus. The latter is an historic route into the pelvis. The old song about Frère Jacques was about a real person, a 'cutter for the stone', who travelled Europe removing bladder stones by inserting his knife and gripping tongs into the bladder through the perineum. He must have had great success, to judge from the numbers of countries whose folklore includes him. The trend today is to use the abdominal route rather than the perineal route.

Very great care is taken not just to remove the whole prostate, within which is the whole cancer, but also to preserve two important functions – urinary continence and the man's power of erection. This means not disturbing the nerves and blood vessels running around each side of the prostate towards the base of the penis, which are essential to erection. If the tumour is close to them, this may not be possible. It also means very careful reconstruction of the structures around the base of the bladder once the prostate is removed, so that the bladder responds normally to the message that it is becoming full, and is able to contain, without leaking, the volume of urine above it. Preserving the 'sphincter' (the muscle that closes around the top of the urethra to shut off the exit from the bladder) in this way is technically very difficult.

Radical prostatectomy has its disadvantages. It is a major operation and even in the best series, published by experienced surgeons who have done virtually nothing else for years, there are occasional unwanted complications. One is urethral stricture, in which the outflow from the bladder is partly obstructed by scarring that leaves the upper part of the urethra too narrow. It can be very uncomfortable, but it can be dealt with relatively easily. One that is more worrying is leakage of urine that can become serious incontinence. There are many fewer cases of incontinence after prostatectomy now that the techniques have become more refined and the anatomy around the base of the bladder is better understood.

In the past, every patient undergoing radical prostatectomy was impotent afterwards, as the nerves to the penis were routinely cut in the removal of the gland. Today, the surgeons know much more about the distribution of these nerves and how they work, and have techniques to identify them and to avoid cutting them. The result is that many men who need to retain their sexual activity can do so, and now that we have sildenafil (Viagra) we can help those who have become impotent, too.

How successful is radical prostatectomy? The latest series of long-term studies of men after this operation show that they survive as long as men of similar age without prostate cancer. It is difficult to beat that! These excellent results stem from the fact that the men undergoing the operations are chosen because they have tumours considered to be curable, and are therefore healthier (and often younger) than men with more extensive disease. The results are also excellent because surgeons are specializing more in this type of surgery, which hones their skills and knowledge. The care immediately after surgery is also better, especially the management of post-operative pain and healing. It is so good, in fact, that the average man stays in hospital only two and a half days after the operation.

Some prostate cancer centres give their patients anti-androgen treatment for some weeks before they perform the radical prostatectomy. Anti-androgen therapy is explained in Chapters 14 and 15, as its main use is in men whose cancers have metastasized before diagnosis, but its principle is that it will shrink the cancers, because the individual cancer cells depend on androgens (testosterone and dihydrotestosterone) for their growth.

Reports on the use of anti-androgens before surgery have been good. The surgeons report that at operation after anti-androgen treatment the prostate is much smaller than it was at diagnosis and that its margins are much clearer. This makes it easier to dissect it away from the crucial nerves and blood vessels that promote erection, and to preserve urinary continence. They also report just as good long-term survival rates as surgeons who operate earlier without a period of anti-androgen therapy. However, the experts are still divided on whether or not to give anti-androgens before surgery. The debate should be settled by two trials, one in Europe and one in North America. They are comparing the long-term survival of men who have had radical prostatectomy with and without previous anti-androgen therapy. So far, there has been no difference between them, but it will be some years before we can compare their long-term survival.

Of course, some men who have had a prostatectomy do develop recurrent cancers later, probably because some small areas of cancer outside the prostate were not recognized, or even detectable, at the time of operation. The first sign of such recurrence is a rise in PSA level, so everyone who has had a prostatectomy for cancer must return for repeated PSA tests for the rest of their life. Around one-third of men whose PSA doubles within six months of their operation may eventually develop a recurrence. This compares with around one in six of men in whom the PSA doubles 18 months after their surgery.

Local recurrence like this may frighten you, but it must be put into perspective. Among ten large studies of men after radical prostatectomy for cancer, the recurrence rate over the next 15 years or so ranged from 8 per cent to a maximum of 31 per cent. In most of the studies, the recurrence rates were around 10 per cent. This is astonishingly good for a cancer operation of any organ, and it has to be considered in the context that even a recurrent cancer can still be treated very successfully by anti-androgen therapy. It is by no means a death sentence. We do not just have one shot at the target: radical prostatectomy is just the first of many treatments we can use.

### Who should be offered a radical prostatectomy?

The accepted expert view today is that it should be the first choice in younger, fitter men whose cancer is localized to the prostate, and who have reasonable expectations of living for at least another ten years. But they must be fully informed about the risks and benefits. One question they may well ask is 'Is radical prostatectomy a better option for me than the "wait and see" policy mentioned at the start of this chapter, or than radiation therapy?'

We do not yet know the answer, but prostate cancer surgeons are faced with having to make decisions for them. Which is why I asked Graham Holland about how he does so.

His wide experience and his knowledge of the results reported worldwide persuade him that radical prostatectomy, external-beam radiotherapy and radon seed therapy (see Chapter 13) have similar complete cure rates. They are all meant to be curative, but there is always the possibility that there are microscopic distant areas of spread not identified at the time of treatment. So a small minority of men do develop detectable secondary spread later. Their numbers don't seem to depend on the type of treatment they have had.

Cryotherapy as a first step may not have the same success rate. It now uses the cold gases argon and helium, rather than nitrogen, and the system is more popular in the USA than in

Europe. Graham Holland would use it only if radiotherapy has not had the expected benefit. He is not convinced that it is as effective as the other choices. He tends to use radical prostatectomy in younger men and radiotherapy in older men. His definition of 'older' and 'younger' did not depend on age but on assessment of the patient's life expectancy. If they are likely to live at least another ten years, he goes for surgery. In those with a shorter probable future, the choice is radiotherapy, but the patient also takes part in the decision.

## Unwanted effects

One aspect of surgery that must be considered when making the decision is the man's quality of life after his recovery. Skilled surgeons like Graham Holland always try to avoid interfering with the nerves that control erection and ejaculation, which run like a fine network over the prostate surface. If they are damaged, even slightly, sexual problems are likely. The more experienced the surgeon, the lower is the chance of them, but sometimes they are inevitable. In fact, Graham told me that almost every man has some difficulties with producing and maintaining erection after radical surgery. Some US surgeons claim post-operation impotence rates as low as 30 per cent, but this may be a matter more of different definitions of impotence here and across the Atlantic. At follow-up in the USA men are asked if they have had any erections after their surgery. If they say 'yes' they are counted as 'not impotent' even though they have not managed full penetrative sex. In Britain any difficulty with erection, maintaining erection and ejaculation is counted as an unwanted effect. The true figures for sexual difficulties after surgery are probably the same for experienced surgical teams on either side of the Atlantic.

If you do have erectile difficulties after surgery you may be given a 'phosphodiesterase type-5 inhibitor', the best known of which is sildenafil (Viagra). Others are tadalafil (Cialis) and vardenafil (Levitra). Your doctor will guide you on which might be the best for you, how and when to take it and its side effects.

A small number of men also become incontinent after surgery – they can leak urine. How serious this is depends on how close the cancer is to the outlet of the bladder and the urethra, and how easy it is to dissect the prostate away from the delicate nerve and muscle mechanisms at the base of the bladder. Before your operation your surgeon will guide you on your particular risks of having these problems afterwards. Remember that if you are being considered for radical prostatectomy that means your surgeon is aiming at complete cure, and he or she thinks that you have an excellent chance. As with impotence, the more experienced your surgical team is, the lower are your chances of having urinary problems.

## Robot-assisted surgery

One last comment on surgical treatment of prostate cancer. Since the first edition of this book a new type of surgery has been devised – robot-assisted laparoscopic prostatectomy. At the time of writing (2010) it is still in its early stages, and surgeons using it are still learning the skills. It is offered in only a few centres in the UK, but it is predicted to be the main form of surgery in the near future. I hope that the next edition of this book will carry more information about it.

# 12

# Radiation therapy

Radiation therapy is another option for men with localized prostate cancer. It is offered to the same men who are offered radical prostatectomy. They have cancer confirmed by biopsy that as far as is known is confined to the prostate.

Radiation therapy has the big advantage of offering a cure without surgery. As prostatectomy is a major operation with all the usual risks, this advantage cannot be underestimated. However, it has its disadvantages. First of all it does not help BPH, so it can leave men with bladder outflow problems that still need treatment, perhaps TURP (see page 45). The radiation can injure the nearby bowel and bladder, so that some men who have had it need operations to repair the damage. A small number have been reported, for example, to need a colostomy (a bowel opening in the front of the abdomen) because the radiation has damaged the rectum.

Radiation treatments take a long time – they need many sessions in the radiotherapy department, which can be daunting. Unlike radical prostatectomy, radiation therapy leaves the prostate behind, so that there is a potential for future cancers to develop, and for men to remain anxious about it. Of course, there is also the objection that, as with radical prostatectomy, the radiation therapy may not be needed, because the tumour will not grow fast enough or spread wide enough to cause serious illness or death.

Reading the two paragraphs above would put anyone off considering radiation treatment, but they should be put in context. Today, before you have any form of treatment, you must be fully informed about its possible disadvantages: this is as relevant to radiation therapy as it is to surgery. That is why everyone considering radiation therapy should know what can go wrong. The converse is that a lot can go right.

The main form of radiation therapy using an external beam, when given to the appropriate men, has excellent survival rates. In major US studies more than half of the men survived healthily for more than 15 years. This is similar to survival after radical prostatectomy and also to the 15-year survival rates in men without known prostate cancer of similar age. In other words, most men who have radiation therapy to their prostate cancer can look forward to living a normal and long life.

Those US figures, published in the early 1990s, relate to radiation treatments given in the 1970s. Today's techniques, in which the radiation beam is much more focused on the tumour itself and causes much less radiation damage to nearby tissues, should offer even better results and many fewer complications than those of a generation ago. The UK ProtecT study (mentioned in Chapter 8) is the most comprehensive comparison of the results of more modern radiation therapy, surgery or 'wait and see'. It involved 1600 men with cancer limited to the prostate. The radiation therapy used in the UK ProtecT trial is a more sophisticated and advanced system – called radical conformational radiotherapy – than was used in the older trials. We can't give a true comparison of the success rates of the three approaches until the final study report is published, probably several years from now.

Nowadays, too, many prostate cancer specialists offer, along with the radiation, surgery to remove possibly affected lymph glands in the pelvis. Such surgery is much less complex and serious than radical prostatectomy, and may 'catch' the few men with early spread that is not detectable under the usual tests.

## After radiation therapy

Once you have had your radiation therapy, what then? You will be under surveillance for the rest of your life. You may be asked to have occasional needle biopsies, and you must have repeated PSA tests, to make sure that the cancer is not returning. The PSA does not fall so fast or to such low levels after radiation as after radical prostatectomy, partly because the prostate gland is still there, and some of the normal cells are still functioning (radiation 'takes out' the cancer cells selectively). However, men whose PSA levels drop below one ng/ml after radiation have a much lower chance of a recurrence than those whose PSA remains above four ng/ml.

## Advances in radiation therapy

### Conformational radiotherapy

Failure rates of around 10 per cent after conventional external-beam radiation have led some centres to use new methods to deliver a higher dose of radiation more accurately and more selectively to the tumour. This is the conformational radio-therapy mentioned above (see page 81), in which a CT scan is used to make a three-dimensional model of the prostate, and the radiation beam is 'shaped' to conform exactly to its outline. This not only appears to be more effective but also leaves fewer and less serious side effects than other radiation techniques. Future radiation plans include different types of radiation to kill the tumour cells, among them 'fast neutrons', protons and photons. Early results suggest that they have high response and cure rates.

### Combination radiotherapy and anti-androgen hormone therapy

Another advance in radiation therapy is its use along with anti-androgen hormone therapy. The combination is thought to have two benefits:

- any tumour cells that survive the radiation cannot multiply because they are being hit by the hormone effect (see Chapter 14 for an explanation); and
- depriving the tumour cells of their androgen stimulus while at the same time exposing them to radiation is a double blow that may well kill them.

The results of trials of this combination of radiation followed by four months of androgen blockade were published by the Radiation Therapy Oncology Group (RTOG) in two large studies. The first study reported that in 93 per cent of the men their tumours were completely eradicated: they showed no recurrence up to at least two years later. The second study compared radiation therapy only versus radiation plus anti-androgen treatment in men with disease that had advanced beyond the prostate into the pelvis. In these men, for whom complete cure is unlikely, by five years the disease had spread in 46 per cent of the men on combined treatment and in 71 per cent of those who had had radiation only. Twice as many men were completely free of their disease in the combined treatment group (36 per cent) than in the radiation-only group (15 per cent) after five years. They may seem low percentages, but remember that they already had advanced disease before they had their treatment.

The European Organisation for Research and Treatment of Cancer (EORTC) compared radiation treatment alone with radiation plus anti-androgen treatment. Over three years there was complete local prostate disease control in 95 per cent of the men given the combined treatment and 75 per cent of those given radiation alone. Eighty-five per cent of the men on the combined treatment were metastases-free, compared with 48 per cent of the radiation-only group.

Figures like these have led to a consensus that all men undergoing radiation treatment for prostate cancer should also have anti-androgen treatment for at least four months afterwards.

## Summary

To summarize the information about treatments for early cancer that has not spread outside the gland into the pelvis or distantly:

- The final decision on whether to offer surgery or radiation, plus anti-androgen treatment depends not just on the cancer specialist, but on you, the patient, and your family.
- The risks and benefits differ from person to person, and you can make an informed decision about whether to go ahead with a particular treatment only if you know all the facts. You may only need to wait and see. You may need surgery or radiation therapy. You probably also need anti-androgen therapy. The decision ultimately depends on the discussion you have with your prostate cancer specialist.
- You cannot make the decision without full information about your particular cancer and the risks and benefits of treatment.

# 13

## Other treatments for localized prostate cancer

Most men with localized prostate cancer who need active treatment, rather than being left to 'wait and see', are treated either with radical prostatectomy or radiation therapy plus anti-androgens, and they do well. However, natural anxieties about the unwanted effects of these treatments have led to the development of alternative treatments with potentially fewer and less severe side effects and with, it is hoped, the same success rate or an even better one.

### Brachytherapy

Probably the most used of these other treatments is brachytherapy. Brachytherapy has a long history, dating from 1909, when Parisian doctors Pasteau and Degrais reported their use of radium capsules, which they planted into the urethra of men with prostate cancer. The capsules were soon replaced by radium needles inserted into the cancers themselves, so that the source of the radiation was inside the tumour, rather than beside it. The technique of inserting sources of radioactivity into the prostate became known as brachytherapy, from the ancient Greek word *brachy*, meaning short – the source was a short distance from the tumour.

Throughout the twentieth century radium was replaced by radioactive iodine (for the technically minded, the isotope used is I-125, the radiation from which has a very short field of activity). Needles containing the correct dose of I-125 could be used to plant 'seeds' of radioactive material at intervals of under 1 centimetre, and this would cover the whole prostate. The aim was to give a higher dose of radiation to the tumour, but a much lower dose to the bladder and rectum nearby. The whole radiation dose is given with one insertion, so avoiding the repeated visits needed for external-beam radiation, and saving the time of hospital staff and patients.

This process sounds ideal, but it had its problems. It was very difficult to 'map' the prostate adequately and to get the distribution of the needles or seeds correct. Some parts of the prostate were overdosed and others underdosed, and long-term follow-up revealed unacceptably high failure rates. When external-beam radiation became much more accurate, brachytherapy fell from favour.

## New methods of brachytherapy

In the early 2000s it was revived by the team in the Northwest Prostate Institute in Seattle, in the USA, led by Drs Haakon Ragde and Michael Brawer. They use ultrasound systems to guide the needles carrying the 'seeds' of radioactive material into exactly the correct sites. Some patients, mainly with low-grade cancers, are given I-125. Others, with cancers that appear more actively multiplying under the microscope, are given palladium-103, a radio-isotope whose radiation disappears faster than that from I-125. It can be given in a much higher dose because the time of radiation is so much shorter, with the result of a greater tumour-kill in men whose cancers are highly active and multiplying fast.

The Northwest team use this form of brachytherapy for men with stage T1 or T2 disease that is thought to be localized to the prostate. Not all men are suitable for it. The needles are inserted through the skin of the perineum. If the prostate is very large, the pelvic bones can make it difficult for the surgeon to place the needles in the ideal pattern. Such men may need anti-androgen treatment first, to shrink their prostate before they can be given their brachytherapy. Most men who have had a previous TURP for BPH are unsuitable for brachytherapy because there is not enough prostate tissue left into which the seeds can be planted correctly. In men at high risk of spread of their cancer, who have large tumours, a high Gleason score, and high PSA levels, the Northwest team first use external-beam radiation and follow it up with brachytherapy two weeks later. The implants are inserted under general or spinal anaesthesia, so that the procedure is painless and even relatively comfortable.

## After brachytherapy

Most men can go home within three hours of their brachy-therapy. They may need standard everyday painkillers for a few hours afterwards, but it is remarkably free of after-effects, except for, perhaps, some blood in the urine. They may need drugs to ease the flow of urine from the bladder for about a month.

In the past, people with inserted radium seeds were excluded from close company for a considerable time, because they were sources of radiation that might be dangerous to others. With modern brachytherapy, the radiation is almost completely con-fined to the prostate gland, so that such precautions are not needed. However, to be absolutely safe, men with seeds inserted should avoid close contact with pregnant women or with young children for two months. They may start having sex again after two weeks, providing they use a condom on the first few occasions to collect any seeds that may have migrated into the semen. Follow-up is the same as for radical prostatectomy and external-beam radiation – after one month, then three-monthly, then annually after 19 months. PSA levels are measured regu-larly and a prostate biopsy is taken at 18 months.

## Results

How do the results of brachytherapy compare with those of radical prostatectomy and external-beam radiation? Dr Ragde and his colleagues reported their results of 147 men given brachytherapy and followed for ten years. Given that they were elderly men to begin with (they ranged from 53 to 92 years old, most being around 70 when they were treated) their results are remarkable:

- 67 were still alive and well, with no evidence of prostate disease.
- 54 had died, but only three of them actually died from their prostate cancers; the rest died from the usual problems associated with old age, quite unrelated to their prostate disease.
- 26 were still living successfully with their cancers in a non-progressive phase.

This means that there were three failures (deaths due to the disease) in 147 men, defined medically as 98 per cent disease-specific survival.

This is a huge success. Of course, some of the survivors still have their prostate cancers, but few of these cancers appear to be life-threatening or to be advancing rapidly. Most of the men, too, will reach old age without having to face death from their cancer. These results are similar to those produced by radical prostatectomy and external-beam radiation. They are yet another reason for men with prostate cancer to be optimistic about the future.

## Cryotherapy

Prostate cancers can be frozen as well as irradiated. Cryotherapy, or cryoablation, the use of freezing probes to destroy prostate cancer, has a history stretching back to 1964. The system uses hollow tubes inserted into the appropriate parts of the prostate under ultrasound guidance, just as with brachytherapy. A mixture of argon and helium gases at very low temperatures is then passed along the inside of the tubes, to create an 'ice ball' at the end. Early use of cryotherapy using liquid nitrogen had led to promising results, but it was difficult to stop the freeze extending to the rectum and bladder, where it caused considerable and permanent damage in a few patients. The substitution of the argon–helium mixture for liquid nitrogen has fine-tuned the freezing technique, so that it is now being regularly used in the USA as an alternative to radiation. However, my local consultant, Graham Holland, in Ayr, told me in 2009 that it is used in the UK only as a second-line treatment when external-beam therapy has failed to produce the desired effects, and even then it is little used in the UK.

## Hyperthermia

If freezing is not satisfactory, is hyperthermia (heating up the prostate) a better alternative? There are reasons, which we need not go into here, for thinking that cancer cells are more susceptible to dying from heat than normal cells, so applying heat to the prostate may kill cancer cells while allowing the normal tissue to survive. The current technique makes use of a probe inserted into the rectum just behind the prostate, the end of which emits microwaves that will heat up the surrounding tissues to around 43 degrees Celsius for around an hour. At least six treatments are given.

It is difficult to be certain how effective hyperthermia is, because all the studies reported so far have combined it with anti-androgen treatment or with radiotherapy, so it is impossible to be sure how much each treatment contributed to the success. In one study of 44 men given hyperthermia with either anti-androgens or radiotherapy, 24 of them had disease that had spread enough to cause severe urinary symptoms. The hyperthermia did not cause any serious side effects and led to a big improvement in their symptoms. Only two of the 27 men showed any worsening of the disease four years later, and nine of the 11 men who had follow-up biopsies were free of the disease.

In another study of men who had a radical prostatectomy between six and nine days after microwave heating had been applied to their prostate glands, the technique missed tumours in certain areas of the peripheral zone, which is the part of the prostate that grows most cancers.

So although hyperthermia had promise, it was not considered a proven reliable form of treatment, and is not used, as far as I know, in the UK.

## Lasers

Laser treatment is a form of hyperthermia, in that the intense light from a laser is converted into heat when it hits the target tissue. A tube is passed into the urethra to the level of the prostate. It delivers, from its 'head', laser light at right angles to its length under guidance from a fibre-optic tube. The surgeons can see exactly where they are applying the light. The result is 'coagulation' (in effect a burn) of tissue to a depth of three or four millimetres. The area removed gradually shrinks into a harmless scar. The technique has mainly been used several weeks after men have had TURP for localized cancer, to 'burn' away any suspected residual prostate cancer tissue.

A 1984 study reported only seven treatment failures among 63 men two years after their laser surgery. Nine years later, another group reported 22 of 26 men as disease-free after TURP followed by laser therapy. However, this was a relatively short follow-up, and none of the men, who all had the initial diagnosis of cancer localized to the prostate, showed the fall in PSA values to near-zero that is needed for reassurance of cure.

New laser techniques are being developed that will surely be used eventually in routine treatment of prostate cancer, but the evidence that lasers are preferable to the tried and trusted treatments for prostate cancer is still sparse. We may have to wait years before we have enough data on it to make a reasoned decision on whether or not it should be used.

# 14

# Cancer beyond the prostate – 'locally advanced' cancer

As mentioned earlier, prostate cancer spreads in two ways. First, it spreads through its surrounding capsule (its outer 'skin'). This is defined as locally advanced prostate cancer, and this chapter deals with the treatment of this type of cancer. Secondly, there is distant spread to other organs, usually bones, called 'metastatic' prostate cancer. Its treatment is described in the next chapter.

Cancers that have spread through the prostate capsule are no longer curable by radical prostatectomy, so it is not an option. There have been a few studies of the use of surgery in men who first have three months of anti-androgen treatment, in an effort to 'down-stage' their cancers from 'locally advanced' to 'prostate only'. There are two objections to this:

- there is little evidence that anti-androgens will completely remove all cancer tissue outside the prostate; and
- subjecting such men to radical surgery does not improve their long-term survival any more than does a medicine-only approach.

External-beam radiation used on its own in such men is also disappointing. Most men in trials of this technique alone for locally advanced cancer showed evidence of residual cancer afterwards. Their cancers also tended to become metastatic, so the men treated in this way had a poorer life expectancy than men offered other treatments. Their PSA levels, too, did not drop steeply enough to give doctors confidence that it is a complete treatment.

These findings led specialists towards devising other treatments for locally advanced cancers. The first was to add anti-androgen treatments to radiotherapy. This approach more than doubles the number of men who remain free of progressive cancer after five years. Adding anti-androgen treatment to radiotherapy reduced the proportion of men whose cancers progressed in the next five years from 71 per cent on radiotherapy alone to 46 per cent.

The second choice is to do without the radiation, and use anti-androgen therapy alone. The decision to drop radiation from treatment in locally advanced prostate cancer comes from studies in which anti-androgen alone has had good results, without the complications that can arise from radiation.

## Anti-androgen therapy

### Oestrogen

The first anti-androgen was the female sex hormone, oestrogen. Giving oestrogen to a man with prostate cancer shuts down the production of testosterone, the main male sex hormone, by the testes. As most prostate cancer cells depend on testosterone to grow and multiply, this arrests the progress of the cancer, and leaves the cells open to 'apoptosis', the process in which cells 'commit suicide'. Oestrogen treatment did ease the symptoms of prostate cancer, but at the expense of feminizing the man, so that he grew feminine breasts, lost all sexual desire, and became impotent. It was a high price to pay for a treatment that in the end was not a cure.

### Castration

Castration, by removing the testes at operation, was introduced in the 1940s. It had far fewer side effects. The prostate gland no longer has the stimulus of testosterone, and without the extra oestrogen, the man does not turn into a pseudo-female.

Castration is highly successful: it checks the growth of cancer, reducing the volume of the growth by more than 60 per cent, and often by 80 per cent in almost every case. For locally advanced cancers inside the pelvis, this means there is much less pressure on the bladder, urethra and rectum. Men who had the operation felt much better within hours of the operation. Their bladder outflow problems, their pelvic and abdominal tenderness, their difficulties with bowel movements and their feelings of general ill-health, were almost instantaneously relieved. The operation itself is a relatively minor one, usually performed under a local or spinal anaesthetic, and causes much less discomfort than radiation. A few men are bruised afterwards, and even fewer have minor infections at the site of the operation, that can be readily dealt with.

Naturally, castration has its major drawbacks, not least the understandable reluctance that any man would feel at losing his testes. After castration, most men lose their sexual feelings and become impotent: in men with a good sex life its loss can seem worse than death itself. And castration is irreversible.

### Drugs that reduce testosterone output by the testes

Happily there are now excellent medical, reversible, alternatives to castration that do exactly the same thing – remove the ability of the testes to produce testosterone. These are drugs that fall into two classes:

- pure anti-androgens; and
- luteinizing hormone releasing hormone (LHRH) agonists.

They need a chapter of their own to describe how they act in the body (see Chapter 15). For the purposes of this chapter, keeping in mind that it is about locally advanced prostate cancer without distant metastases, they can be used instead of castration, and have the benefit of being able to be used in intermittent 'bursts' of treatment. The most commonly used anti-androgen drugs for locally advanced cancers are bicalutamide (Casodex), flutamide (Drogenil), leuprorelin acetate (Prostap), goserelin (Zoladex), and buserelin (Suprefact).

Why should they be used intermittently? Some researchers believe that giving anti-androgens constantly to men with locally advanced cancer may increase the risk that the cancer cells may become able to multiply in the absence of androgens. In medical terms they become 'androgen-independent', and therefore much more difficult to control. Androgen-independent cancers no longer respond to anti-androgen treatment, and need different types of chemotherapy. It would be far better to avoid this development. One way to do this is to deprive the cancer of androgen enough to drive the PSA level below four ng/ml, and to keep it there for 32 weeks. The man should then be considered for stopping his anti-androgen treatment at the 36th week.

Over the next eight to 14 weeks his testes will start to work again, and his testosterone level, and his PSA level, will gradually climb until they are back to their pre-treatment figures. The general rule is that if the man's PSA level is under 20 ng/ml at first diagnosis, then the next course of anti-androgen drugs is started when the PSA has returned to that first measurement. If the initial PSA was above 20 ng/ml (and it can be in the thousands), then the next course of anti-androgens is started when the PSA (having fallen to near zero after the first course of treatment) has returned to 20 ng/ml.

This second course of treatment continues until the PSA has fallen again to near zero, and carries on for another 32 weeks before the treatment is again stopped. The next cycle of treatment is again started only after the PSA has risen, as after the first cycle. Many patients go through five or more of these treatment cycles with no evidence of any advance in the tumour, and most show real shrinkage of their cancers.

These repeated courses of anti-androgen therapy interspersed with periods of no treatment have several advantages. They may prevent cancers from becoming androgen-independent and therefore resistant to treatment. Just as important, they improve the man's quality of life. Stopping the drugs causes any side effects to disappear. The men recover their sexual feelings (that are almost always lost on anti-androgens), they feel generally better, and they are protected to some extent from one common complication of deprivation of androgens, the 'brittle bone disease' osteoporosis. It is difficult to know for sure that intermittent anti-androgen therapy is better than constant anti-androgen therapy. The only evidence so far is a small trial in which the long-term results were similar to those of continuous androgen deprivation.

## Treating the complications of locally advanced prostate cancer

When prostate cancers enlarge and spread into the neighbouring tissues, they tend to cause two major complications:

- bladder outflow problems; and
- pressure on the ureter (the tube from the kidney to the bladder).

Bladder outflow problems in any man are far more likely to be due to BPH than to locally advanced cancer, and the usual treatment is TURP (see page 45). However TURP often leads to urinary incontinence (mainly constant leakage of urine) when it is done for cancer, rather than for BPH. Most prostate specialists would therefore prefer to shrink malignant obstructions with anti-androgens instead of operating. Unhappily for the men, while they are on this treatment they need to be catheterized (with a permanent drainage tube from the bladder to the penis). One way to avoid this is to place a 'stent' (a small section of tubing) inside the urethra to keep the narrowed section open. Most people do not notice that their stent is in place, and can urinate normally, but some find it painful and uncomfortable, and it can lead to bladder infections. Stents can also move upwards into the bladder or downwards and out during urination, so they need close supervision while they are in place. After around three months, when the prostate has shrunk enough for normal urination to resume, the stent can be removed.

Stents can also be inserted into an obstructed ureter for the same reason – pressure by an expanding tumour or by nearby enlarged lymph glands on the back of the bladder. If it is impossible to do this, the next step is to bring the affected ureter out on to the abdominal wall, so as to ease the back-pressure on the kidney on that side. This is called a nephrostomy.

Very rarely (thankfully, because it is a miserable condition) prostate cancers grow locally so large that they wrap themselves around the bowel behind them, making the man extremely constipated and uncomfortable (he feels as if he is always needing to empty his bowel, but cannot, no matter how he strains). Although anti-androgen treatment may help these men a lot, some finally need a colostomy (a bowel opening on the front of the abdomen) to give them relief.

# 15

# Cancer beyond the prostate – metastatic disease

By the time prostate cancer has spread distantly, with metastases in bones and other organs, surgery is no longer an option. First and foremost, if the multiple tumour sites are to be hit hard, the man needs 'androgen ablation' – the removal of all influence that androgens such as testosterone exert on the tumour cells. As is the case for men with cancer that has spread only within the pelvis (see Chapter 14), the options are either castration or the use of anti-androgen drugs, and this is probably the right place to describe how the two main types of anti-androgen drugs work.

## LHRH agonists

The first group to be developed were the LHRH agonists (the initials stand for luteinizing hormone releasing hormone). LHRH agonists are drugs that cause the pituitary gland to pour out LHRH into the bloodstream. LHRH is a confusing name for the hormone in men, because the name relates to its action in women. Another, probably more appropriate, name for LHRH is gonadorelin, so that LHRH agonists are also called gonadorelin agonists.

To understand how LHRH agonists work, one must know a little about the way the pituitary gland regulates the release of sex hormones by the ovary and the testis. Luteinizing hormone (LH) is released by the pituitary gland (which hangs down from the base of the brain inside the skull) into the bloodstream. In women LH is released mainly in mid-menstrual cycle, and it causes the ovary, in turn, to release the hormone progesterone into the bloodstream, and to 'drop' an egg into the uterus, ready for fertilization. If conception takes place, then the progesterone prepares the lining of the womb to receive the fertilized egg by initiating the first stages of the formation of the placenta, the organ through which the developing infant is nourished and by which it is anchored to the womb. In the meantime the spot on the surface of the ovary from which the egg has fallen becomes the corpus luteum (Latin for 'yellow body'). The corpus luteum produces the hormone human chorionic gonadotrophin (hCG), which then sustains the pregnancy by helping it to firmly embed into the wall of the womb.

Luteinizing hormone (LH) was therefore named in this way because it led to the formation of the corpus luteum. It was only later discovered that exactly the same pituitary hormone is used in men to cause the testes to produce testosterone. Without the message of LH from the pituitary, the testes produce no testosterone, and the man is 'medically castrated'.

Now we have to go one step back in the biochemical chain. LH is produced by the pituitary only if it is told to do so by another hormone, produced by an area of brain just above it called the hypothalamus. This hormone is called LHRH – luteinizing hormone releasing hormone – for the elementary reason that it causes the pituitary to release LH into the bloodstream, from which the testes pick up the message to produce testosterone.

### How do LHRH agonists reduce testosterone levels?

So far, so good. But why give an LHRH agonist if you wish to stop the testes from producing testosterone? Logic suggests that it will make the testes produce more testosterone, not less. That is true. Give an LHRH agonist to a man and there is a fast rise in testosterone levels to around 150 per cent of normal. But within 21 days of starting continuous treatment with an LHRH agonist, testosterone levels plummet to near zero, to the levels seen after castration. This is because constant exposure to LHRH switches off the pituitary's response, and it no longer produces

LH. The testes have no stimulus to produce testosterone, so it stops producing it. And it will not start producing it again until the LHRH agonist treatment is stopped.

## Examples of LHRH agonists

As with locally advanced prostate cancer (see Chapter 14), the LHRH agonists used for metastatic cancer include buserelin (Suprefact), goserelin (Zoladex), leuprorelin acetate (Prostap) and triptorelin (Decapeptyl).

- Buserelin is unique among them in that in long-term use it is delivered by nasal spray. For the first week it is given by three daily injections under the skin: then the man changes to the spray, giving himself six sprays a day from then on.
- Goserelin is given by a solid rod implant, delivered through a wide bored needle, under the skin of the front of the abdomen. It can be given as Zoladex once a month or as Zoladex LA once every twelve weeks.
- Leuprorelin is given as an injection of 'microspheres' through a syringe under the skin either as Prostap SR once a month or as Prostap 3 once every three months.
- Triptorelin is also given as a microsphere injection of Decapeptyl sr, once every four weeks. Microspheres are tiny spheres containing the drug, designed to release a steady amount of it into the surrounding tissues over the month between injections.

LHRH agonists must be given in these ways because when they are swallowed they are digested and therefore would not work.

## Direct anti-androgens

The second type of anti-androgen includes cyproterone acetate (Cyprostat), bicalutamide (Casodex), and flutamide (Droganil). There is also nilutamide (Anandrone), which is not in use in the UK. These direct anti-androgens do not work on LHRH.

Instead they block the formation of testosterone by the testes and of dihydrotestosterone by the adrenal glands. As mentioned in Chapter 3, the adrenal glands, which sit above the kidneys, produce a small amount of androgen.

## Using both types of anti-androgen together

Now comes the difficult bit: how can these two types of anti-androgen be used to the maximum benefit of men with metastatic prostate cancer? There is no argument among the experts on the first way in which they are used – on the day of diagnosis and for the next three weeks. However, the experts are keenly (even fiercely) divided on how they should be used after that.

The main aim of the initial treatment of metastatic prostate cancer is to remove the influence of testosterone as fast and as effectively as possible. However, just giving an LHRH agonist alone would mean exposing the man to a week or so of higher, rather than lower, blood levels of testosterone, before they began to fall. This can make the symptoms worse for a while, as the cancer cells become more active. It can lead to more intense bone pain, and make the man feel more ill. If he has a metastasis in one of his vertebrae, the consequent swelling can put pressure on the spinal cord. Such spinal cord compression can lead to weakness and paralysis, so it must be avoided at all costs.

These increasing symptoms immediately after starting men on LHRH agonists is called a 'flare', and it can last up to three weeks.

The flare phenomenon is why, for those first three weeks, men with metastases at the time of diagnosis need both types of anti-androgen. Either cyproterone acetate or flutamide is given along with the LHRH agonist. They prevent the initial rise in testosterone that LHRH agonist would cause, so avoiding the flare. Then, as the long-term effect of the LHRH agonist 'kicks in', the direct anti-androgen can be stopped.

This is where the controversy starts. What should be done next? The argument revolves around whether the direct anti-androgens should be continued, along with the LHRH agonist, or whether it is better for the LHRH agonist to be given on its own. Some experts believe the two should be continued together, to make sure that even the smallest amount of androgen in the blood, including both testosterone and the androgens made in the adrenal gland, is abolished. This 'maximal androgen blockade' has been pioneered by Dr Fernand Labrie and his colleagues in Quebec. Dr Labrie is a real enthusiast for the dual treatment, and it is only fair to say that I have been present at meetings in which the debate for and against his methods has been spirited, to say the least.

His argument goes like this. Just blocking the androgen (testosterone) produced by the testes using an LHRH agonist leaves untouched the androgen (DHT, or dihydrotestosterone) that is produced by the adrenal glands. Dr Labrie and his colleagues say that the adrenal androgen may still stimulate prostate cancer cells, and that this stimulation should be switched off by adding a direct anti-androgen such as flutamide to the LHRH agonist. They say that the combined drugs give a better initial response in more men, delay the time to the tumour developing androgen independence (see Chapter 14), lengthen the time to the cancer starting to increase again (defined as cancer progression), and improve survival rates.

The argument against Dr Labrie's approach is that giving both types of drug together over long periods increases the patients' side effects and is a considerable extra cost. These objections may not be too important if the combination of the two types of drug does actually improve life quality and length of survival, but are very important if it does not. So it is incumbent on supporters of Dr Labrie's management to prove that it does what is claimed for it.

Have they proved their point? It is still difficult to say, although recent studies are increasingly suggesting support for them. The Quebec team's first published study, in 1985, showed such good figures on combined treatment that they were hardly believed by the other prostate cancer researchers at the time. Only one of 87 patients with metastatic cancer died within two years of the diagnosis, and only eight of the cancers had progressed. These figures are considerably better than comparable studies using LHRH agonists alone, and they led to many more studies being undertaken.

Some of them tended to support the Quebec team, but others found no difference in survival, or in time to recurrence of the disease, between the combined treatment and the use of LHRH agonists alone. It must be admitted that almost all of the trials showed that the two-pronged attack on the cancer led to a longer delay to signs of recurrence of the cancer, but not necessarily to a longer life. When the Prostate Cancer Trialists Collaborative Group (PCTCG) examined 22 trials involving 5710 men, the estimated risk of death was between 6 and 22 per cent lower with maximum androgen blockade than after castration alone. Although surgical castration is not the same as LHRH agonist treatment alone, it has a very similar effect.

One way to judge treatment effectiveness is to measure the PSA levels. When 411 men were treated either with leuprorelin plus placebo or leuprolide plus flutamide, 76 per cent of the men on the two drugs, but only 52 per cent of the men on leuprolide plus placebo, reached normal PSA levels within three months. This is fairly strong evidence that the combination may be more effective in shutting down cancer activity.

Where do I stand in the debate? First of all this is my own opinion, not necessarily the correct one, and probably not one shared by most prostate cancer consultants. It has been formed from what I have read and from conversations with cancer specialists, and not from personal experience of treating hundreds of men with prostate cancer. A GP like me will only see a few new cases per year, so any judgement from my own experience can only be anecdotal. For what it is worth, however, if I have the misfortune to have the disease myself, and it is metastatic from the start, I would wish to have maximum androgen blockade, with (at the moment) flutamide and one of the LHRH agonists. My view may change as trial results are published in the future. Many consultants still hold to the view that adding a direct anti-androgen to LHRH agonist treatment is only adding side effects, and not extra life or quality of life. I fully respect that decision, and would ask men faced with the decision on management of their tumours to discuss the difference between the two treatments, and their relevance to their special case, openly with their consultant. There may be good reasons for either treatment in any individual case.

### What is the position in the UK?

In the UK, the official position is that LHRH agonists are licensed for use alone for metastatic prostate cancer and that the direct anti-androgens cyproterone acetate, flutamide, and bicalutamide are licensed for use in preventing flare in the first three weeks of LHRH agonist treatment. Cyproterone acetate and flutamide are also licensed for use on their own as treatment for prostate cancer that has progressed on LHRH agonist treatment. So far, bicalutamide is licensed only for locally advanced, non-metastatic cancer, and not yet for metastatic cancer. This may change as the results of current large trials of its use in metastatic cancer are eventually reported. In any case, each prostate specialist is free to prescribe what he thinks is needed by each patient.

## Side effects of anti-androgens

If you read the list of side effects on the inserts inside the packages of the various anti-androgen drugs, you will probably be shocked at their number and severity. However, do understand that this is an extensive list covering every side effect that has been reported, and that most of them are rare. Side effects that are not rare, however, are the ones that are caused by the drugs' main actions, such as testosterone suppression.

LHRH agonists, because they have such strong effects on hormone levels, produce symptoms very similar to menopausal problems in women. Common ones are hot flushes, drenching sweats, loss of sexual desire and impotence. Much less common are rashes and itch and, even more rarely, asthma and severe allergic reactions. Some men have a red, swollen, irritating reaction around the injection site. Other very occasional reactions include headache and migraine, hair loss, dizziness, muscle and joint pains, swelling of the ankles, indigestion, weight changes (either up or down), difficulties in sleeping and swings in mood.

Taking direct anti-androgens along with LHRH agonists can heighten all these symptoms. They may also add a risk of liver problems, including jaundice, abnormal heart rhythms, a tendency towards diabetes, pain in the pelvis, anaemia and bleeding disorders. Nilutamide, for example, can make it more difficult for you to adapt your vision quickly when going between light and dark environments, and it can lower your tolerance to alcohol.

Cyproterone acetate differs from other direct anti-androgens in that it is a 'progestogen'. When given over many months the testes overcome its ability to suppress testosterone formation, so that testosterone levels tend to rise again. As its side effects include an increased risk of thrombosis (blood clots in veins) and a tendency to induce diabetes, as well as to cause liver problems, it is used only for short periods unless it is a last resort when all else has failed.

## When androgen suppression fails

There are times when LHRH agonists and direct anti-androgens have failed or are no longer appropriate, or when they need supporting by other drugs. One drug that is used widely to 'shrink' prostate tissue in BPH, finasteride (Proscar), may find a use in men with prostate cancer, too, provided that it is always given with, rather than instead of, an anti-androgen. Many men have both BPH and prostate cancer, and there is some evidence from animal studies that it may have anti-tumour activity as well as the ability to reduce benign overgrowth of prostate tissue. In one trial in men who had residual prostate cancer after radical prostatectomy, giving finasteride delayed the subsequent rise in PSA by about 18 months. When given with flutamide it was as effective in keeping rises in PSA at bay as goserelin plus flutamide. At present, however, finasteride is not recommended officially for prostate cancer: whether that will change depends, as is usual with new uses of drugs, on the results of ongoing trials.

## Summarizing management of metastatic prostate cancer – the picture in 2010

The first line treatment for prostate cancer that has spread to distant sites is to remove androgens either by castration or by using LHRH agonists. The trend is away from surgical castration towards 'medical castration' with LHRH agonists, with the proviso that in the first three weeks a direct anti-androgen is used to prevent flare. Many specialists use maximal androgen with both an LHRH agonist and a direct anti-androgen long term, particularly in fitter and younger men in whom it could be expected that they could live long enough eventually to die with, rather than from, their cancer. In older men there may be good reason to use an LHRH agonist on its own, to minimize the side effects that are commoner on the two-drug system.

I wrote in the first edition of this book that there is optimism that the near future will bring drugs that can be taken by mouth that will not only avoid the need for surgery or injections, but also allow men taking them to have a normal sex life. Sadly, by 2010 they haven't arrived.

Sadly, too, if you already have metastatic cancer you don't have the choice of 'wait and see' described in the previous chapter. That policy is confined to cancers that have not spread beyond the limits of the prostate. Once the cancer has spread, LHRH agonists with or without a direct anti-androgen are needed to deal with the symptoms and to prevent further spread of the disease.

# 16

## Dealing with androgen independence

Unfortunately there sometimes comes a time when even expertly treated prostate cancers become androgen-independent. Despite continuing complete androgen blockade, the cancer begins to spread again, and further anti-androgen and LHRH treatment no longer helps. The first sign of this development is a rise in PSA despite continuing low testosterone levels. Sometimes, paradoxically, this rise is arrested and even reversed by stopping the anti-androgen therapy. Experts in the field believe that this is because some of the cells have mutated, so that they are now stimulated, rather than stunned by the anti-androgen. So the first action in someone taking, for example, flutamide plus an LHRH agonist and whose PSA is rising, is to stop the flutamide. That may be all that is needed to slow or stop the cancer progressing.

If that action fails, then the next step is to use one of two different approaches. One is to use drugs that increase oestrogen levels in the blood. There is some evidence that oestrogen will directly harm prostate cancer cells. One oestrogen used in this way is the oestrogen diethylstilboestrol (DES). It may keep the cancer at bay for many months, but only at the price of side effects such as the development of feminine breasts. It is also linked to deep vein thrombosis and heart problems, but these can be prevented by taking just 75 mg of aspirin a day.

A more complex oestrogen that is more often used in metastatic prostate cancer is estramustine (Estracyt). It combines in one capsule oestrogen and mustine, an anticancer agent.

Estramustine seems to concentrate in the pr
it selectively destroys cancer cells, and
that around 60 per cent of men given it after i
androgen treatment respond well to it, by feeling
around half of them there is also good objective evidence
the tumour has responded. Unfortunately, estramustine can
also affect the bone marrow, so that it can cause anaemia and
damage the white cells. It also may cause nausea that does not
easily respond to anti-nausea drugs. If any of these side effects
occur, it has to be stopped.

Studies of other cytotoxic (anticancer) drugs in prostate
cancer that has become resistant to anti-androgens have been
disappointing so far. The National Prostate Cancer Project
(NPCP) in the USA has published a series of trials of different
combinations of cytotoxic drugs, among them cyclophospha-
mide, 5-fluorouracil, streptozotin, hydroxyurea, vincristine, and
cisplatin along with estramustine. The response to them has
been mixed, sometimes only a little better than the response to
placebo.

## Palliation

There comes a time in the life of some prostate cancer patients
when the aim is not necessarily to keep the cancer at bay, but
to ease the symptoms that it causes. This is described as pallia-
tion, and the symptom that most needs it is bone pain. Bone
pain from cancer deposits may well not respond to the usual
painkillers, whether they are based on aspirin, paracetamol or
morphine.

However, it may respond to bisphosphonates. These are
drugs designed originally for women with osteoporosis, where
the bones are losing calcium. Bisphosphonates are a group of
drugs that direct calcium into bones and prevent calcium loss
from them. They are used successfully in bony metastases from

east cancer. As long ago as 1985 an injectable bisphosphonate, clodronate, was reported to ease bone pain in 16 of 17 men given it for androgen-independent prostate cancer. Newer bisphosphonates given by mouth may be as effective. When the bone pain is localized to one spot, radiotherapy can help a lot, given as a single dose or over several weeks. More extensive bone pain may be treated with wide-field radiotherapy, in which half the body is irradiated in one dose, then the other half later. Unfortunately, wide-field radiotherapy is extremely debilitating, with more than a third of men receiving it feeling sick and having diarrhoea. It is reserved for men whose bone pain is very severe and who may wish to take the risk. It does relieve the pain completely in around 30 per cent of the men treated, and another 50 per cent report at least a partial response.

One form of radiation treatment, strontium-89, has been useful for bone pain. It is taken up preferentially where there are particularly active metastases, shutting down the bone activity, and relieving the pain. A review of several studies reported relief of bone pain in 78 per cent of men given it. Others have shown similar results. A British study in 284 men also concluded that men given strontium-89 were less likely to develop new sites of pain than others given external-beam radiotherapy.

Strontium-89 produces milder side effects than other forms of radiotherapy and cytotoxic drugs: it is given as a single dose, and its effects usually last three months or more. After that time more doses can be given if the need arises.

If the worst happens, and all treatment eventually fails, then care must be put into the hands of a team of carers experienced in palliative care, and the patient's relatives and his GP should be involved. The aim of all treatment is to try to prevent the patient reaching this final stage, but it is only common sense to plan ahead. Most men naturally wish to stay at home for as long as possible, but there are times when a move to a nursing home is the sensible thing to do. It is best to organize a move like this in advance, so that the transfer is not done in a rush into a place that may not be to your liking. If this is the case for you, please heed your doctor's and nurse's advice. It may not seem like it, but is usually the best for you: the main aim at this stage is to keep you comfortable, and the most likely way for this to happen is under the care of experienced professionals.

# 17

## Coping with sex

This subject has been left until now, not because it is the least important, but because sexual activity can be a problem at any stage of prostate cancer and its treatment. It is one thing to be treated successfully for prostate cancer, but quite another to have treatment that preserves the enjoyment and mechanics of a normal sex life. Men today are open about the need to preserve the quality of their sex lives, and, it follows, of their partners' sex lives, too.

It has to be accepted that treatments for prostate cancer do interfere with your sex life. The old operation to remove the prostate in men with early cancers divided the nerve and blood vessels to the penis, so that sexual feelings and erection were both lost, for good. The newer operations, which go to great lengths to spare both nerves and blood supply, have greatly improved the chances that after healing both sexual feeling and potency will be normal. Nevertheless, only about half of men undergoing modern radical prostatectomy return to their full sex lives afterwards.

TURP is more successful in maintaining both sexual feelings and potency, but even with this operation, in which the material removed is not near the nerves and blood supply to the penis, around 16 per cent of men have subsequent problems with starting or maintaining an erection, or both. Why this happens is not clear. All forms of radiation therapy, including brachytherapy, may also lead to impotence, mainly because the arteries within the prostate, which lead to the penis, are affected by the radiation. Studies suggest that around 60 per cent of men remain potent with normal sex lives after external-beam radiation therapy.

Brachytherapy seems to be better at preserving potency: of 56 men in one brachytherapy study, 85 per cent of them were still potent after three years. On the other hand, cryotherapy has a bad record: 88 per cent of 74 men undergoing cryotherapy, who had had a normal sex life before treatment, were impotent afterwards.

Castration (which is used less and less these days as a treatment for prostate cancer) reduces sexual desire in most men, and with it comes impotence, but not in all men. Presumably their potency depends on the androgens produced by the adrenal glands (see page 21). 'Medical castration' induced by maximal androgen blockade (that is, the use of an LHRH agonist plus a direct anti-androgen) causes a complete loss of interest in sex and impotence because it removes even the small amount of androgen produced by the adrenal glands. In an Italian study, taking goserelin and cyproterone acetate together led to 86 per cent of the men becoming impotent and losing interest in sex.

Most men, obviously, would like to retain their normal sex lives, despite the danger of a slightly higher risk of dying from their disease. This is one reason put forward for giving bicalutamide to some men with advanced cancers who wish to keep on enjoying sex. Bicalutamide is the drug, so far, that is most successful in maintaining potency in men with advanced prostate cancer. However, it is not as good as other drugs in treating metastases in bone. This is a trade-off that is difficult to measure, and should be a matter for serious discussion between patient and specialist.

Impotence can be treated without the need to put you at greater risk of cancer spreading. Today, you can learn to inject materials such as the drug alprostadil into the penis (using Caverject or Viridal) or into the urethra (MUSE – Medicated Urethral System for Erection) to produce an erection. You can use a vacuum device, or take one of the Viagra-like pills. Eighty per cent of 15 men with problems with erection after a radical prostatectomy found success with sildenafil.

Some men remain potent and have orgasms after prostate surgery, but no longer ejaculate. This is commonest after TURP, when the ejaculate goes into the bladder, rather than out through the urethra. Anyone having prostate surgery, whether it is for BPH or cancer, should be warned beforehand that this may happen. Many men who find that this is happening avoid sex: if they are warned beforehand they and their partners can usually cope. Attempts to correct the backward flow of sperm after surgery have met with little success: with guidance and advice, most men accept it as an inconvenience, rather than a disaster. The sperm is expelled with the next urination.

In the very small number of men with prostate cancer who still wish to father children, sperm can still be obtained by applying an electrical current to the nerves and blood vessels around the remaining prostate gland tissue. Whether this is desirable, considering the doubts about the future health of the father, is an ethical, not a medical, matter.

# 18

## Some general comments

In health matters, the USA is often the trend setter. Since American doctors started to use PSA as a detection tool in the 1980s, far more prostate cancers than ever before have been detected in their curable early stages. Because of this, and because treatments are more effective, the numbers of deaths from prostate cancers have actually declined in the USA – an astonishing fact, considering that there are so many more older men than there used to be.

PSA tests have helped enormously to pick up the early cases before they reach stages for which cure is impossible. There may be new tests that will detect the cancers that are most likely to metastasize early and that need more urgent treatment. One of them may be measurement of blood levels of E-cadherin (see page 24). Another may be the identification of genes that increase the chances of prostate cancer in families in which there have been several cases. Already two such genes are known. However we are years away yet from using that knowledge to treat disease.

New radiotherapy techniques may be developed that will pick out and treat only prostate cancer cells, leaving normal tissues undisturbed, and avoiding incontinence afterwards.

Another idea is chemoprevention, in which drugs given to men at potential risk of prostate cancer may prevent it from developing. Two candidates for this are similar to vitamins A and D. Another is finasteride, mentioned previously, which is already widely used to reduce prostate size in BPH. Further ahead are possibilities for gene therapy, and the use of genes to enhance the body's own immune defences against cells that are beginning to turn into cancers.

Another possible way forward is to prepare 'vaccines' from chemical products of the man's own cancer cells and induce an immune response against them.

I mention all these approaches (and there are many more) to show that research into prostate cancer is expanding fast in many directions. Two or three of them will surely be significant forward steps in its diagnosis and treatment. Looking back, it is amazing how far we have come in the past ten years or so.

Since 2006 I have written the 'Doctor, Doctor' column in the *Guardian* Saturday magazine. In it I answer questions from readers, and I am struck by how many of them ask about ways that they can help themselves to keep healthy and prevent disease. Most of them relate to how much exercise they can do and what they can eat to lower their chances of preventing or living longer with diseases like cancer. Some have been from men at high risk of, or who already know that they have, prostate cancer.

It is difficult to give them a positive answer. As far as we know, there is no relationship between different diets and prostate disease. The common belief that eating foods or taking supplements containing anti-oxidants has not been borne out by rigorous and large trials, some of which even showed that people taking such supplements have a higher early death rate than control subjects who were given placebo. There is some suggestion that vegetables and fruits containing lycopenes, such as tomatoes, apples and green tea, may protect against cancers, but that has not been linked specifically to prostate cancer.

As for exercise, people who take regular exercise usually feel better, and that has to count as a benefit. One set of exercises, often used by women after giving birth, aims to strengthen the pelvic floor. They can be useful for men who have surgery or radiation in helping them to retain bladder control. Mr Holland, my consultant colleague in Ayr, recommends them. Your physiotherapist will be glad to teach them.

Most important, if you have prostate cancer, please get in touch with The Prostate Cancer Charity. This is an excellent organization that works with and for you. It funds research, provides support and information, and is constantly campaigning to improve your life and the lives of men like you. The charity has a confidential helpline manned by specialist nurses – 0800 074 8383. It is open during weekday office hours and also from 7 p.m. to 9 p.m. on Wednesdays. It has produced a pack of information that includes *Prostate Cancer: A Guide for Newly Diagnosed Men*, and a tool kit information pack about the disease. You can order them from <literature@prostate-cancer.org.uk>, and you can download all their publications from the website at <www. prostate-cancer.org.uk>. All the charity's materials are accurate, very readable and up to date.

Other important websites are:

- <www.dipex.org.uk>, in which men who have prostate cancers share their experiences;
- <www.goingfora.com>, a virtual hospital set up by the Royal College of Radiologists, in which staff and patients share with you information on scans and cancer treatments;
- <www.prosdex.com>, which is an aid to men who wish to know whether or not they should have their PSA level measured; and
- <www.cancerscreening.nhs.uk/prostate>, which is an NHS website showing why there is no national screening programme for prostate cancer, and leading you into the NHS informed choice programme.

I highly commend all these sites. People with cancer have never been better informed than now, and that is especially true of prostate cancer.

# Index